D1038264

# EDUCATING RNS FOR THE BACCALAUREATE:
## Programs and Issues

**Barbara Klug Redman, Ph.D., M.S.N., B.S.N.,** is executive director of the American Nurses' Association. Dr. Redman received her B.S.N. from South Dakota State University, and her M.S.N. and Ph.D. from the University of Minnesota. She has been a Veterans Administration Administrative Scholar and a postdoctoral fellow at Johns Hopkins University. Her professional experience includes serving as assistant dean at the University of Minnesota School of Nursing, dean at the University of Colorado Health Sciences Center School of Nursing, and executive director of the American Association of Colleges of Nursing. During her tenure as executive director of AACN Dr. Redman oversaw the activities of the Baccalaureate Data Project.

Dr. Redman has published extensively on patient education and different aspects of nursing education, including curriculum revision. Her book, *The Process of Patient Teaching in Nursing*, has been translated into Japanese and Finnish and is in its sixth edition. She has served on the editorial boards of numerous journals, including *Journal of Nursing Education*, *Patient Education and Counseling*, and *The Diabetes Educator*.

**Judith Mary Cassells, D.N.Sc., M.S.N., B.S.N.,** provides consultation on nursing ethics and teaches at the Georgetown University School of Nursing. Dr. Cassells is also curently serving as a research clinical assistant on a federal grant, assessing the physiological, psychological, and social needs of patients with AIDS. Dr. Cassells received her B.S.N. from Villanova University and her M.S.N. and D.N.Sc. from the Catholic University of America. In 1983, she was appointed director of the American Association of Colleges of Nursing's Baccalaureate Data Project. Dr. Cassells served as director for both phases of the Project, which focused on expanding the national database for generic students (Phase I, 1983–1986) and RN students (1986–1988).

Dr. Cassells has developed an interest in ethics as it relates to curriculum design in nursing and supports the development of ethical decision-making skills of students and practicing nurses. She is an elected member of the Advisory Council for the Society of Health and Human Values and an associate member of the Kennedy Institute of Ethics. She is active in many professional organizations, including the Washington DC Nurses' Association AIDS Education Committee. The Committee is providing ongoing education on AIDS for practicing nurses in the DC metropolitan area.

183225

# Educating RNs for the Baccalaureate: Programs and Issues

**Barbara K. Redman,**
Ph.D., R.N., F.A.A.N.

**Judith M. Cassells,**
D.N.Sc., R.N.

*Editors*

REMOVED FROM THE
ALVERNO COLLEGE LIBRARY

610.73071
E24

**Ruth Lamothe**
*Managing Editor*

An American Association of Colleges of Nursing Book

SPRINGER PUBLISHING COMPANY • NEW YORK

Alverno College
Library Media Center
Milwaukee, Wisconsin

The views expressed in this book reflect those of the authors and do not necessarily reflect the official views of the American Association of Colleges of Nursing.

Copyright © 1990 by Springer Publishing Company, Inc.

All rights reserved

No part of this publication may be reproduced, stored in a retrieval system, or transmitted in any form or by any means, electronic, mechanical, photocopying, recording, or otherwise, without the prior permission of Springer Publishing Company, Inc.

Springer Publishing Company, Inc.
536 Broadway
New York, NY 10012

90 91 92 93 / 5 4 3 2 1

---

**Library of Congress Cataloging-in-Publication Data**

Educating RNs for the baccalaureate : programs and issues / Barbara K. Redman, Judith M. Cassells, editors : Ruth Lamothe, managing editor.
    p.  cm. — (Springer series on the teaching of nursing : v.  12)
    Includes bibliographical references.
    ISBN 0-8261-7210-5
    1. Nursing—Study and teaching (Higher)—United States.
  I. Redman, Barbara Klug.    II. Cassells, Judith M.    III. Lamothe, Ruth.    IV. Series.
RT79.E34  1990
  610.73'071'173—dc20                    90-9533
                                                CIP

---

Printed in the United States of America

# Contents

# Preface

One of the challenges of higher education in the 1990s will be continued and expanded adaptation to diversity. Over the past 20 years, the profession of nursing has successfully integrated registered nurses originally prepared with a diploma from a hospital school of nursing or with an associate degree in nursing into programs leading to the bachelor of science in nursing (BSN). During the last decade, there has been a positive response from the nursing education community to the RN population's demand for academic and professional development.

Most observers are aware of the statistics about the increasing average age of college students and about the work that must be accomplished in attracting and retaining minority students. Other diverse groups must also be accommodated. Nursing's experience with integrating this diverse group of RN students into baccalaureate programs can be instructive to the nursing and to the higher education community.

Today, RN/BSN education is tremendously diverse and rapidly changing. Little comprehensive and comparative information has been available about the variety of baccalaureate programs in nursing that admit RN students. Comparisons with generic baccalaureate nursing education on such issues as recruitment, career and educational goals, and student reaction to their nursing preparation and personal development during the educational process would be useful to educators, administrators, and policy makers.

This information is critical to meeting the health care needs of the nation for several reasons: (1) the baccalaureate program is the only RN preparation that incorporates preventive health care skills and knowledge; increasingly, these skills are essential for meeting health care goals; (2) the baccalaureate program is the only RN preparation that prepares for community practice, which is essential for achieving efficient health care expenditures; and (3) the movement of RNs into baccalaureate education is increasing at a dramatic pace and has tremendous potential in determining whether professional-level nursing services are available in various regions of the country.

Recognizing that the face of baccalaureate nursing education is changing rapidly to accommodate new student populations and determining the need for clear, comprehensive information about RN/ BSN programs and the role this information could play in affecting the quality of nursing education and health care, the American Association of Colleges of Nursing (AACN) felt that a comprehensive study of RNs returning for the baccalaureate would be a useful contribution to the literature and could encourage greater exploration of options developed to assist them. This book grew out of that study.

The investigative structure was in place for the Association to conduct such a study, since the first major piece of an overall project to examine baccalaureate nursing education recently had been completed. This first piece, the Generic Baccalaureate Data Project, funded by the Division of Nursing, HRSA, provided extensive data on generic baccalaureate nursing education, including a follow-up of students 6-months and 12-months postgraduation, which added further insight to their perceptions of the educational process and its application to their practice. The Project generated numerous publications: several articles were published in the **Journal of Professional Nursing**, and the final report was widely disseminated and put into the ERIC database.

A book-length format was deemed more useful in disseminating the findings of the second piece of the Baccalaureate Data Project— the RN Baccalaureate Nursing Data Project—because so little well-researched information was available on the RN/BSN population. In addition, the number of RNs returning for the baccalaureate will continue to increase, at least for the next several years, so a careful reporting of this population's characteristics and educational experience would provide a helpful blueprint for educators and administrators who are considering the development of an RN/BSN program. The commissioned chapters were chosen to make the data-based materials from the study more accessible to those exploring the development of an RN/BSN program, and to provide thoughtful commentary from nursing service on the movement of RNs returning to school for the baccalaureate.

This book then, reports on and extends beyond AACN's national survey of BSN education for registered nurses. Sometimes characterized as a movement, the considerable increase in the number of RNs pursuing baccalaureate education has taken place within a historical and political context. Structure and processes of RN/BSN education are described, as is the transition of the new graduates back into the workplace and into graduate education.

The authors provide a set of observations about how both higher education and health care have molded the system for RN/BSN education, and about issues that remain to be addressed. A nurse administrator's perspective is included, and development of a program is discussed in depth from a public and a private institutional perspective. Different educational models serving this diverse population are presented.

The data in this book are from the RN Baccalaureate Nursing Data Project (Grant No. D10 NU23-72), funded by the Division of Nursing, Bureau of Health Professions, Health Resources and Services Administration, Department of Health and Human Services Administration, Department of Health and Human Services.

# Acknowledgments

Without the effort of a strong, diligent advisory committee, many projects would founder and produce reports that have little or no impact. The RN Baccalaureate Nursing Education Data Project was gifted with a hard-working, incisive committee whose members are gratefully acknowledged.

**Thelma L. Cleveland, R.N., Ph.D.**
Dean
Intercollegiate Center for Nursing Education

**Sylvia E. Hart, R.N., Ph.D.**
Dean
University of Tennessee-Knoxville
College of Nursing

**Joan M. Hrubetz, R.N., Ph.D.**
Dean
St. Louis University
School of Nursing

**Judy M. Strayer, R.N., Ph.D.**
Chair
Otterbein College
Department of Nursing

**Judith Lewis, R.N., Ed.D.**
Director
California State University
Statewide Nursing Program

**A. Susan Nelson, R.N., Ph.D.**
Chair
Corpus Christi State University
Baccalaureate Nursing Program

**J. Mae Pepper, R.N., Ph.D.**
Chair
Mercy College
Department of Nursing

Auxiliary staff, who were anything but, are also gratefully acknowledged:

**Sarah C. Haux, M.S.**
Project Coordinator

**Susan S. Jackson, R.N., M.S.N.**
Research Associate

**Rita Furst Seifert, Ph.D.**
Statistical Consultant

# Contributors

**Judith Balcerski, R.N., Ph.D.,** is Dean of the College of Nursing, Barry University, Florida, a post she has held since 1969. Dr. Balcerski served on the American Association of Colleges of Nursing Taskforce, which authored *Essentials of College and University Education for Professional Nursing*. Dr. Balcerski holds a Ph.D. in Higher Education Administration from the University of Michigan, a M.S.N. from Wayne State University, with a major in the Administration of Nursing Education Programs, and the B.S.N. from Barry University.

**Geraldine (Polly) Bednash, R.N., Ph.D.,** is Executive Director of the American Association of Colleges of Nursing, Washington, D.C. Dr. Bednash serves on the Editorial Board of *Nursing Economics*, and is a reviewer for the *Journal of Professional Nursing, Image*, and *Nursing Economics*. Dr. Bednash holds a Ph.D. in Higher Education Policy and Law from the University of Maryland. She has been a Robert Wood Johnson Nurse Faculty Fellow in Primary Care at the University of Maryland. She received the baccalaureate in nursing from Texas Woman's University, the Master of Science in nursing from The Catholic University of America. Dr. Bednash is a member of Sigma Theta Tau. Dr. Bednash coauthored the groundbreaking study on the costs and benefits of nursing study which was published as a monograph, *The Economic Investment in Nursing Education: Student, Institutional, and Clinical Perspectives*.

**Maryann F. Fralic, R.N., M.N., Dr.P.H.,** is Senior Vice President, Nursing, Robert Wood Johnson University Hospital, New Brunswick, NJ, and Clinical Associate Dean, Rutgers University College of Nursing. Dr. Fralic is a member of the editorial boards of *The Journal of Nursing Administration, Nursing and Health Care, Nursing Connections*, and is a reviewer for *The Journal of Professional Nursing*. Dr. Fralic is a Fellow in the Johnson & Johnson–Wharton Fellows Program in Management for Nurses. She is a national and international consultant, and author and lecturer in Health Care and Nursing Administration. Dr. Fralic holds a doctorate in Health Services Administration.

**Dorothy L. Powell, R.N., Ed.D.,** is the Dean of the Howard University College of Nursing, Washington, D.C. Prior to coming to Howard, Dr. Powell served for 11 years as chairperson, Department of Nursing, Norfolk State University, Norfolk, VA. Other positions held include Assistant Professor, Maternal-Child Nursing at George Mason University, Fairfax, VA, Hampton University, Hampton, VA. She also served as chair of the associate degree program at Thomas Nelson Community College, Hampton, VA for four years. Dr. Powell holds an Ed.D. in Higher Education Administration from the College of William and Mary, Williamsburg, VA, an M.S. in Maternal Infant Nursing from Catholic University, Washington, DC, and a B.S. in Nursing from Hampton University, Hampton, VA.

**Alma S. Woolley, R.N., M.S.N., Ed.D.,** is Professor and Dean of the School of Nursing, Georgetown University in Washington, D.C. She received her B.S.N. from the Cornell University School of Nursing, her M.S.N. in medical-surgical nursing, and her Ed.D. from the University of Pennsylvania. Dr. Woolley has worked as a public health nurse in New York City and as a staff nurse in New York and Philadelphia. She has taught nursing at the University of Pennsylvania and at Atlantic Community College. She was the Carolyn F. Rupert Professor of Nursing and Director of the School of Nursing at Illinois Wesleyan University in Bloomington, IL, from 1981 to 1986. Dr. Woolley has served as an N.L.N. accreditation visitor and as a member of the Board of Review. She is a member of the Editorial Board of *Nurse Educator* and is a member of the board of directors of the A.A.C.N. She has written and published particularly in the areas of nursing education and nursing history.

# EDUCATING RNS FOR THE BACCALAUREATE:
## Programs and Issues

# 1

# Introduction

There is an apparent movement underway in nursing education: Increasing numbers of registered nurses (RNs) prepared with associate degrees in nursing and diplomas from hospital schools of nursing are enrolled in programs to earn the bachelor's degree (BSN) in nursing. Note the following evidence: (1) in 1985, RNs comprised 32% of bachelor's degree students; (2) between 1975 and 1984 the number of RNs enrolled in bachelor's degree programs that also admit generic students (students with no previous nursing education) increased by 11%; (3) the number of bachelor's degree programs that admit RNs only rose to a high of 170, and the number of RNs enrolled in those programs almost quadrupled; and (4) the number of RNs graduating from baccalaureate programs increased from 3,763 in 1975 to over 10,000 annually by 1984 (Rosenfeld, 1986). In 1985–86, more than 46,000 RNs were enrolled in programs to achieve the bachelor's degree (NLN, 1988).

Clearly, such figures are evidence of a movement in one sense of the word. What is less clear is how long this flow of students will last and whether the increase in RN/BSN education represents a growing concurrence that obtaining a first level of education and later adding to it is to be a permanent or favored structure in nursing education. Indeed, the numbers could be interpreted as a movement toward favoring professional education in nursing on the part of both students and employing agencies.

This book describes RN/BSN education as it exists in the

United States today. It seeks answers to questions of student motivation in returning for the degree, of student satisfaction with the programs, and of the early postgraduation career development of graduates. It also provides information about issues that have been sensitive—access to programs, geographic, economic, and time-related—and credit transfer and validation experiences of current senior students. Descriptions of program design, coursework completed by RN students for the BSN, and progression through the program have not been available until now.

Understanding how the profession has adapted to the needs of the increasing number of RNs returning for the BSN is important for nursing educators and administrators. We suspect that the education system has entered a new phase of this accommodation, reflecting the results of experimentation and learning, and that satisfying experiences may be had in programs reflecting the several different structures that accept RNs for the BSN.

In truth, there were few examples in higher education to imitate. Whereas most other professions have upgraded the preparation of their workers during this century, few other professions have had the diversity of basic preparation opportunities for their practitioners. Efforts to upgrade the basic preparation of all professional nurses and/or to provide opportunities for enhanced education for the basic practitioner prepared outside the baccalaureate education model is a massive educational extension for nurses. In addition, lack of differentiation of technical and professional roles in the work places in which these individuals had served for years has further confused the issue. Individuals prepared for basic nursing practice through either diploma, associate degree, or bachelor's degree programs are most often employed similarly, with similar work role expectations and salaries.

As a result, nursing educators needed to fashion an appropriate experience for RN students working toward a BSN, using the general concepts of articulation, psychology of adult learning, and delivery of education to adult populations that are found in various sectors of higher education. Such a baccalaureate program also needed to take account of previous learning, life and work experiences, and the additional elements of basic professional nursing education to be included.

What is presented here are data about RNs' baccalaureate educational experiences and the structures in which they occur; comparison, when possible, to prior data; and inspection of the differences and similarities among the program structures. The study on which this book is based does not provide information on how many capable and motivated RNs feel they have access to this BSN education or how well the health care industry takes advantage of the additional education RN/BSNs bring to the workplace, especially more than a year after completion of the degree. It also cannot predict how conditions in the marketplace, including salaries, will act as incentives or disincentives to attaining the BSN or whether there will be further state regulation requiring articulation between ADN/diploma and baccalaureate nursing education.

The return of RNs to school to earn the BSN has been a positive step, but it also presents some challenges. It means that a larger percentage of nursing personnel is available to function in roles requiring this level of preparation. What will be the response of the health system? Many observers feel that a richer mix of professional to technical personnel is badly needed for the future as well as for the present. "Based on current trends, by the year 2000, there will be roughly one half as many baccalaureate and higher degree nurses and 1⅓ times as many ADN/diploma nurses required to meet a nursing personnel need conservatively estimated at 858,800 FTE baccalaureate nurses" (DHHS, 1987). To meet this identified need, the output from baccalaureate programs should be doubled (Styles & Holzemer, 1986). It is important to note also that, on the average, hospitals would like to have 55% of their RN staff prepared at the baccalaureate level. At present, an average of 20% of full-time staff RNs are baccalaureate-prepared; nearly every respondent hospital surveyed by the American Hospital Association (AHA) desired a more highly educated staff (AHA, 1987). This is an impressive showing of support for the qualities that a university education in nursing can provide.

At the same time, the increase in numbers of RNs returning for the BSN also requires a considerable investment in accommodating structures for individuals with very diverse academic preparation in the liberal arts and nursing and experience in the field. At present, this cost is primarily borne by baccalaureate programs. The costs associated with articulation include development of special curricular options, provision of challenge opportunities, alternative class-scheduling opportunities, and a host of other factors. In general, upper-level programs have been expected to provide mechanisms for transition of students prepared in these 2- and 3-year programs. It has been acknowledged that articulation assumptions and arrangements represent a political position and that there are many ways in which they can be structured (Stevens, 1981). Stevens comments that articulation assumptions are based on differing views of the realm of knowledge that is included in either the "so-called technical or so-called professional programs." Obviously, articulation models or arrangements will differ based on the educator's views regarding the knowledge specific to each level of nursing education.

Therefore, it is useful to understand how the present system came to be and to view this movement in the context of the effect on nursing education of policy and institutions from both the health and the higher education sectors.

## HISTORY OF BACCALAUREATE EDUCATION FOR RNS

Before 1950, few RNs went on for degree study. At that time there were 200 nursing programs leading to the bachelor's degree and another 1,000 leading to a diploma (Searight, 1976). Shane (1983) has described three eras of RN/BSN education:

1. The years—1909 to 1960—when a second form of nursing education was established. Although RNs could be asked to start at the beginning of the freshman year and complete everything, including the nursing, to earn the baccalaureate in fact most schools required RNs to complete only the general education courses. There was wide variation in the amount of credit awarded for completion of the diploma program and in the techniques for determining which and how many credits were to be awarded for the diploma. Many schools offered specialized programs in nursing education or nursing administration at the baccalaureate level for RNs.

2. A middle era—1960 to 1972—began when the NLN adopted a policy that there should be a single generalist nursing program leading to the bachelor's degree for both generic and RN students, some upper-division courses in nursing should be required

of all students, and blanket credits for diploma nursing courses were outlawed.

3. The present era—1972 to the early 1980s—has been noted for establishment of upper-division programs for RNs only. As indicated earlier, programs grew rapidly during this time. The first nurses were graduated from associate degree programs in 1954. Based on the premise that the functions of technical nursing could be differentiated from those of professional nursing, associate degree programs were specified as complete in themselves, preparing the graduate for immediate employment (Montag, 1980). These programs grew rapidly, and thus, even in a period of decline of diploma education in nursing, the presence of associate degree programs ensured an ongoing concern about upward mobility into professional nursing of individuals prepared for technical nursing. One has to assume that this pressure was in part related to the fact that graduates from all three kinds of programs were eligible to take the RN licensing exam.

It must be understood that these developments took place against a history of transition from apprenticeship education—a form of education that shares many commonalities with other professional fields of study such as medicine. Apprenticeship education, with its focus on craft methods, practical experience, and limited theoretical education, was characteristic of the hospital school of nursing. In the case of medicine, however, 19th-century philanthropic foundations gave their funds and, perhaps more important, the support of a sponsoring elite to reshape and empower medical education to became professional. Nursing education never enjoyed this level of support. This observation is based on the view that professions are not just special organizations of work but particular expressions and vehicles of dominant class and culture (Melosh, 1982).

Since the end of the 19th-century, there had been a small core of nursing leaders who pushed reform, the goal being professionalization. During World War II, nursing leaders moved decisively to increase the number of baccalaureate-prepared nurses and to establish more collegiate programs. By the end of the war, the outlines of today's nursing education were visible. The Brown report of 1948 (Melosh, 1982) boldly asserted the goal of baccalaureate education for nursing, although even as late as 1971 diploma schools graduated more new nurses than did AD and baccalaureate programs combined.

Finally, external developments overcame the apprentice model of education. Nurses needed more theoretical training to meet the demands of work precipitated by advances in health science in World War II, and a theoretical education also facilitated adaptation to the rapid changes that followed. Further, hospitals began to increase their concerns about the costs associated with support of diploma schools of nursing and began to close these schools as access to other education increased for potential nursing students. Since World War II, educational and professional opportunities for women have opened up significantly. Thus, nursing, seen traditionally as a woman's profession, has been pushed into competition with the other opportunities.

Melosh (1982) believes that this history has left nursing with two difficulties. First, nursing's elite leaders were unwilling to undertake the task of upgrading nurses already in practice. The consequence of that choice was in part nursing's persistent internal conflict over the movement to professionalism. Second, she makes the observation that the culture of apprenticeship continues to reproduce itself on the job. In truth, both the traditions of professional ideology and the apprenticeship culture provide resources for moving toward nurses' claims to authority at work (Melosh, 1982).

The work of the National Commission on Nursing Implementation Project (NCNIP) (1987) projects a transition by the year 2000 to two clearly differentiated nursing roles—technical and professional—and addresses the issue of differentiated use of these products in the health care system. The diagram and accompanying text in Appendix A (at the end of this chapter) describe timelines for the transition and imply that the new technical degree and the new professional degree will be different from those of today. Included in NCNIP's work is development of new practice models that provide a framework for application and testing of differentiated nursing roles based on different educational experiences. These models should also provide a framework for continued refinement of the RN/BSN educational experience.

## OTHER INFLUENCES

RN/BSN education is, of course, influenced by the external environment in both education and health care and in particular by the labor market for nurses. Literature comparing practices in 12 fields of professional education found nursing to be highly influenced by its professional community. It also found a strong belief that technical competence deserves considerable emphasis, a concern with professional socialization experiences intended to develop identity with the professional role, and a tendency to organize and closely supervise field experiences (Stark, Lowther, & Hagerty, 1987). One could surmise that this focus is in part an expression of the apprenticeship culture.

RN/BSN programs also reflect general practice in universities regarding interinstitutional credit transfer and articulation agreements. Indeed, conflicts between professional fields and community colleges concerning these matters are not limited to any particular field. The American Association of Collegiate Schools of Business is reported to have established standards that specify that an undergraduate school of business should concentrate its professional courses in the last 2 years of a 4-year program, leading to difficulty with transfer of business credits from the associate of applied business degrees (Savage, 1986).

In several states, the matter of articulation between AD/diploma education and bachelor's degree education has been the subject of legislation. In 1979, the Arkansas legislature enacted a law requiring nursing schools in that state to accept previous credits or develop challenge exams, mandating that RNs should be able to attain 60 credits toward the bachelor's degree by use of these mechanisms. The law apparently precipitated an increase in enrollment of already licensed nurses but not an increase in credits transferred or challenged by these students (Thomas & Thomas, 1987).

In Maryland, political pressure from RNs who felt their access to BSN programs was not adequate resulted in a governor's order to establish a statewide articulation model (Rapson, 1987). The plan required implementation of three options: (1) an advanced placement option, which had been offered by Maryland baccalaureate schools before the model was mandated; (2) transition courses in scientific concepts, social sciences and humanities concepts, and nursing concepts, to be offered for 3 years for RNs prepared in Maryland before 1979 (students taking all three courses earned 60 college credits toward the BSN); and (3) direct transfer of course credits by approval by a committee of the transferring program instead of the individual student. Enrollment of RNs in BSN programs has increased since the plan was implemented.

There are many factors in the employment setting that would affect the decisions of RNs to attain the BSN. In recent years, there has been the perception that the BSN would enhance one's job options and job security (Rapson, 1987). Yet monetary return for the investment in attaining a BSN has been minimal: in 1984 it was estimated to be an average of $1,370 per year over the salary of an AD-prepared nurse. In addition, after 15 years of experience, AD nurses were just as likely to be in higher-level jobs as were BSNs (Link, 1987). Especially in a time of nursing shortage, one would have to wonder whether the strong movement toward the BSN will be reversed as RNs with less preparation find that jobs are plentiful; although the expression of support by nurse executives for a more educated nursing staff could continue the increased enrollment of RNs in baccalaureate nursing programs.

## REVIEW OF SELECTED LITERATURE

Recent literature on RN/BSN education is scattered and partial in its description. It provides information on socialization of RN students as well as several case examples of states that have established systems of outreach to provide BSN education for RNs in rural areas.

Extensive efforts made to provide BSN programs for RNs in rural areas have been described in two states. North Carolina mounted such a program through its Area Health Education Center (AHEC) system. AHECs were conceived by federal legislators as a mechanism for enhancing the availability of health professions education and health care services to rural areas.

In North Carolina, this system has been established to improve the quality, quantity, and distribution of health professionals in the state, operating through links between universities and nine AHEC centers throughout North Carolina. It has been able not only to coordinate the needs of RNs in one area of the state to obtain the BSN but also to provide part of the funds necessary to launch the program (McGrath, 1984). Nebraska has made such programs available at several sites in the state. A cooperative agreement between the University of Nebraska, three state colleges, and four community colleges provided opportunity for RNs to complete nonnursing required and elective coursework. The university offers nursing content on off-campus sites by video- and audiotapes, telephone, conferences, and on-site clinical practice and conferences. Locations for course delivery change from semester to semester and are scheduled according to the number and location of schools (VanHoff, 1983).

Baccalaureate programs have operated on the belief that RNs originally prepared in ADN and diploma programs needed development in professional roles, an understanding of the health care system, and a different approach to delivery of nursing care (Smullen, 1982). Bridge courses are frequently designed to facilitate the transition, focusing especially on the conscious, continual application of theory from many fields to practice and on the autonomy and independent judgment necessary for the professional nursing role. Such courses also provide a socialization function for returning RNs by which they meet and form their own peer groups (Woolley, 1978). (See Chapter 5 for a more detailed discussion.)

Several studies address orientations and concomitant career motivations of students. Little and Brian (1982) gathered longitudinal data from students in six second-step programs (upper-division programs for RNs) and found student types differentiated by their contrasting nursing styles as well as diverse sociopolitical views and personality characteristics. Some students entered the program with images of nursing that were close to "professional," that is, that nursing is not a task-oriented occupation but a profession with intellectual challenges. For some students, the decision to return to school was precipitated by an attempt to move away from technical nursing and to escape the traditional hospital role; others found comfort in the security of authority. Those already on the road to professional nursing before they returned to school made greater gains in intellectual skills and changed more of their attitudes about the health care system. Students who came in still maintaining a more traditional view of nursing made fewer changes and solidified their views on many social issues related to nursing. The authors conclude that it may be too simplistic to assume that nurses are divided into a dichotomy of technical and professional. Stevens (1981) also identifies models for portraying the overlap or separation of professional and technical nursing knowledge and comments that the diversity of educational enterprises available may not ever allow simple delineation of these two concepts. She comments that any attempts by educators to deal with this dichotomy should be based on an ability to articulate the separation of these two realms.

Jako (1983) described several different orientations of RN students. Those with inpatient and community orientations had well-established roles related to providing service and care. Those in the vertical-mobility group valued advancement in the institution and influence and authority. Those in the academic-orientation group valued teaching, research, and the acquisition and dissemination of knowledge. Those identified as frontiering emphasized the importance of moving into new nursing roles and into different modalities of practice. Socialization of students in the BSN program differed according to personality factors and on their preexisting professional identity. Jako challenges the common assumption that all postlicensure students are mature and experienced, especially noting that the 2 + 2 program type, in which an upper-division nursing program is affiliated with an AD program offered through the same institution, had young, inexperienced students.

## THE STUDY

The study of baccalaureate education in nursing for RNs on which this book is based was carried out as a companion to a study of generic baccalaureate education in nursing, which has been reported elsewhere (Cassells, Redman, & Jackson, 1986a, 1986b; Redman & Cassells, 1985; Redman, Cassells, & Jackson, 1985). The Special Report of the Baccalaureate Nursing Data Project is available in the ERIC Clearinghouse (RN Baccalaureate Nursing Education [1986–1988] Special Report. ED299866). Thus, the opportunity is available for comparison between the educational programs for these two populations on elements such as the following:

- institutional setting
- resources available to the program
- faculty qualifications and teaching assignments
- student recruitment
- coursework taken
- student perception of growth and satisfaction with the program
- how the student's education was financed
- career goals, including interest in graduate education
- postgraduation employment on follow-up

Special questions relating to BSN education for RNs include the following:

- types of programs
- jurisdiction of the state board of nursing over the program
- length of time for completion
- scheduling options and outreach programs
- number of credits attained by transfer and by advanced placement
- comparison of work position pre- and post-BSN

The universe of baccalaureate programs offering BSN education for RNs was identified ($N = 606$). The deans of the schools were asked to respond to a survey questionnaire about their programs; response rate was 76% ($n = 461$). For RN students, eligibility was based on a selected birth month of the year. If no students were born during the designated month, the dean used a random numbers table for student selection. Through these efforts, 1,089 eligible students were identified; usable response rate was 68%. Data were gathered during February and March 1987, with student follow-up data gathered during August through October 1987. Response rate to the follow-up survey was 61% ($n = 456$).

The questionnaires were developed by the American Association of Colleges of Nursing (AACN) with input from a project advisory committee and other nursing experts and consultants. The questionnaires were field-tested for content validity, conciseness, and comprehensiveness of information needed. *The Essentials of College and University Education for Professional Nursing* (AACN, 1986), endorsed by the members of AACN, was used in developing the curriculum areas of the questionnaire.

The measurements used included descriptive statistics; percentiles, distributions, measures of central tendency; standard deviations; cross-tabulations using chi-squares; *t* tests between matched and independent groups; and analyses of variance. Whenever possible, regional- and school-characteristic comparisons were done on variables to differentiate between types of baccalaureate programs.

Baccalaureate education for RNs has grown in layers over a period of many decades. There now are a large number of institutions that admit RNs for the BSN. They represent several structural approaches with a variety of articulation methods. A description of the demographics of these programs, students, and faculty may be found in Chapter 2.

## REFERENCES

American Association of Colleges of Nursing. (1986). *The Essentials of College and University Education for Professional Nursing.* Washington, DC: Author.

American Hospital Association. (1987). *Report of the Hospital Nursing Personnel Survey.* Chicago: Author.

Cassells, J. C., Redman, B. K., Haux, S. C., & Jackson, S. S. (1988 April). RN Baccalaureate Nursing Education (1986–1988) Special Report. ERIC Clearinghouse, #ED299866.

Cassells, J. C., Redman, B. K., & Jackson, S. S. (1986a). Generic baccalaureate nursing student satisfaction regarding professional and personal development pre-graduation and one year post-graduation. *Journal of Professional Nursing, 2,* 114–127.

Cassells, J. M., Redman, B. K., & Jackson, S. S. (1986b). Student choice of baccalaureate nursing programs, their perceived level of growth and development, career plans, and transition into professional practice; a replication. *Journal of Professional Nursing, 2,* 186–196.

Department of Health and Human Services (DHHS). (1987). *The Sixth Report to the President and Congress on the Status of Health Personnel in the United States.* Washington, DC: Division of Nursing, Bureau of Health Professions, Health Resources and Services Administration, Department of Health and Human Services.

Jako, K. L. (1983). Orientations toward professional nursing: Traditional to frontiering. In D. L. Shane, (Ed.), *Returning to school: A guide for nurses*. Englewood Cliffs, NJ: Prentice-Hall.

Link, C. R. (1987). *A labor economist's analysis of nursing*. Unpublished manuscript.

Little, M., & Brian, S. (1982). The challengers, interactors and mainstreamers: Second step education and nursing roles. *Nursing Research, 31,* 239–245.

McGrath, B. J. (1984). Completing the BSN off-campus. *Nursing Outlook, 32,* 261–263.

Melosh, B. (1982). *The physician's hand: Work culture and conflict in American nursing*. Philadelphia: Temple University Press.

Montag, M. L. (1980). Looking back: associate degree education in perspective. *Nursing Outlook, 28,* 248–250.

National Commission on Nursing Implementation Project. (1987). *An introduction to timeline for transition into the future nursing education system for two categories of nurse*. Milwaukee, WI: Author.

National League for Nursing. (1988). *Nursing data review: 1987*. New York: Author.

Rapson, M. F. (Ed.). (1987). *Collaboration for articulation: RN to BSN*. New York: National League for Nursing.

Redman, B. K., & Cassells, J. M. (1985). Generic baccalaureate nursing programs: Description of administrative structure and student recruitment practices. *Journal of Professional Nursing, 1,* 172–181.

Redman, B. K., Cassells, J. M., & Jackson, S. S. (1985). Generic baccalaureate nursing programs: Survey of selected enrollment, administrative structure/funding; faculty teaching/practice roles and selected curriculum trends. *Journal of Professional Nursing, 1,* 369–380.

Rosenfeld, P. (1986): *Nursing student census with policy implications*. New York: National League for Nursing.

Savage, D. (1986). Collision course: Two-year colleges and the AACSB. *Community, Technical and Junior College Journal, 57*(2), 48–50.

Searight, M. W. (1976). *The second step: Baccalaureate education for registered nurses*. Philadelphia: F. A. Davis.

Shane, D. L. (1983). *Returning to school: A guide for nurses*. Englewood Cliffs, NJ: Prentice-Hall.

Smullen, B. B. (1982). Second-step education for RNs: The quiet revolution. *Nursing and Health Care, 3,* 369–373.

Stark, J. S., Lowther, M. A., & Hagerty, B. M. K. (1987). Faculty perceptions of professional preparation environments: Testing a conceptual framework. *Journal of Higher Education, 58,* 530–561.

Stevens, B. J. (1981). Program articulation: What it is and what it is not. *Nursing Outlook, 29,* 700–706.

Styles, M. M., & Holzemer, W. L. (1986). Educational remapping for a responsible future. *Journal of Professional Nursing, 2,* 64–68.

Thomas, K. J., & Thomas, H. K. (1987). Legislated articulation of credits: Initial impact of mandated career upward mobility in Arkansas nursing programs. *Journal of Nursing Education, 26,* 78–81.

VanHoff, A. M. (1983). An off-campus second-step BSN program. *Focus on Critical Care, 10*(3), 50–53.

Woolley, A. S. (1978). From RN to BSN: Faculty perspectives. *Nursing Outlook, 26,* 103–108.

**APPENDIX: NATIONAL COMMISSION ON NURSING
IMPLEMENTATION PROJECT**

An Introduction to:

# 1. Timeline for Transition into the Future Nursing Education System for Two Categories of Nurse

# 2. Characteristics of Professional and Technical Nurses of the Future and their Educational Programs

The following pages which describe future nurses and their educational programs have been prepared by the Governing Board of the National Commission on Nursing Implementation Project. These materials reflect a compilation of data from a variety of sources, and represent the input of nurse educators, nurse administrators, nurse practitioners and nurse researchers (see bibliography). Information collected by this project was subjected to review and discussion by Work Group I—Education, for the purpose of identifying the direction nursing was taking across the country. Based on the Work Group review, drafts of the characteristics of professional and technical nurses of the future and a timeline for transition were developed and forwarded to the project Governing Board.

Using a consensus-building process, the board has produced these documents to present a broad view for moving nursing education from four types of educational programs to two. The Governing Board recommends juxtaposing this broad view with complementary national, regional and state documents.

## Use of These Documents

The "Characteristics of Professional and Technical Nurses of the Future and Their Educational Programs" are broad descriptions of educational and practice differences of future nurses. These descriptors, along with national statements on Scope of Practice, state nurse practice acts and organizational job descriptions provide a full picture of nursing in any given setting.

As clients' needs for nursing change and as the knowledge base and practice for nursing adapt to meet those needs, each of the component parts that describe nursing is reevaluated and updated. Such is the dynamic nature of a professional. The "Timeline for Transition into the Future Nursing Education System for Two Categories of Nurse" graphically depicts the change process that has been in effect and projects the completion of the process through the year 2000.

## TIMELINE FOR TRANSITION INTO THE FUTURE NURSING EDUCATION SYSTEM FOR TWO CATEGORIES OF NURSE

The Timeline for Transition into the Future Nursing Education System for Two Categories of Nurse graphically projects (1) nursing education programs today and their transition into the 21st century and (2) a timeline which reflects changes that have been in process and the timing needed to complete the process while maintaining an adequate supply of qualified nurses.

As noted on the timeline, there are presently four types of preparation leading to two types of licenses to practice nursing. Today, preparation for LPN or LVN licensure is currently at the vocational level. Preparation for RN licensure includes the associate degree program with a two-year completion, the diploma program, a three-year course of study usually associated with a hospital, and the college programs offering nursing preparation at the baccalaureate, master's, or doctoral level.

Predictions of the future suggest that there will be dramatic changes in the nature and intensity of nursing care to be delivered. Expansion of technology, a multiplicity of health care settings providing care, and an increase in the aged population with needs for multisystem care, will all affect the type of nurse who will be needed. It is within this framework that the two categories of nurse will evolve from that which now exists.

The expectation that two categories of nurse will evolve from the present four is based on the socioeconomic health care picture that calls for the creation of more cost-effective systems of education. At present the four types of educational programs for nurses are costly because the system prepares nurses in programs with significantly different outcomes and varying levels of ability. These graduates are then employed in a health care delivery system which uses them as if their abilities are the same. The consumer is unaware of the qualifications of the nurse caring for him/her, and the health care system is often not using each nurse to the level of his/ her ability. An educational system which consists of four programs that prepare four categories of nurse, only to provide care either as a registered nurse or a licensed practical nurse, is not cost-effective from either the educational or service perspective. The current nursing education system is inefficient and inadequate to meet future health care needs.

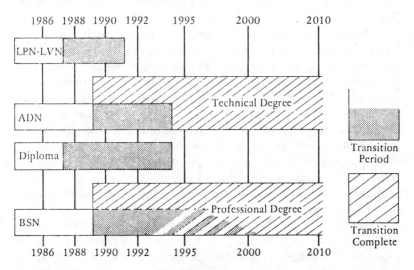

**Figure 1.1.** Timeline for Transition into the Future Nursing Education System for Two Categories of Nurse

## Description of the Timeline

The graph entitled "Timeline for the Transition into the Future Nursing Education System for Two Categories of Nurse" (Figure 1.1) illustrates systematic transition from the present nursing education system to a nursing education system of technical and professional programs for the future. It identifies timelines for transition or closure of programs, including time for curriculum development and transfer of resources while maintaining an adequate supply of nurses. These timelines are approximate, recognizing that transitional periods will vary from state to state.

According to the plan, licensed practical/vocational nursing programs are expected to continue their transitions. Programs now in existence will determine the best use of their resources. This may include developing an associate degree program or closing the program and diverting the resources to another nursing education program. The transition period also allows time for nursing faculty to seek advanced education, if needed, and to prepare for teaching in other programs. The transition of licensed practical/vocational nurse programs is expected to be completed by 1992.

Diploma programs in nursing are expected to continue the transitional phase that has been underway for many years. The timeline projects the conclusion of this process before the end of the century. Present programs will determine the best use of their resources. It is recognized that these programs have a proud history of preparing nurses for their communities. The strengths of these programs should be considered when determining the best mode of change. For some, transition to an associate degree or baccalaureate program in cooperation with a junior or senior college may be feasible. For others, use of the clinical resources and faculty by associate or bachelor's degree programs may be an option.

Present associate degree programs will determine the best use for their resources. The plan for transition will allow for present programs to design curricula to prepare the technical nurse, as described in "Characteristics of Technical Nurses of the Future." In other instances, depending upon the institutional resources and mission, nurse educators may see a need to phase out an associate degree program and develop a program leading to a baccalaureate or graduate degree in nursing.

The transition reflected in the timeline will require national and regional coordination to assure that the changing needs of clients and health care systems will be met by qualified nurses. The transition period will afford nursing faculty the time and opportunity to seek advanced degrees where necessary.

The professional educational programs of the future will be different than the baccalaureate programs of today. The timeline for transition allows time for the present educational programs to design curricula to prepare the professional nurse of the future as defined by the needs of the practice setting and reflected in the "Characteristics of Professional Nurses of the Future."

It is possible that additional time and degrees beyond the baccalaureate may eventually be required for education of professional nurses as described by the future professional nurse characteristics. Some baccalaureate programs may choose to refine and extend their programs to develop those characteristics more fully in their students. Some schools may choose to institute generic master's or doctoral programs.

Critical to any change in the nursing education programs of this country is the assurance that nurses, particularly professional nurses, will be prepared in sufficient numbers to meet the nation's needs. It is imperative that an adequate supply of professional and technical nurses be maintained according to need projections and that individuals are allowed an opportunity to advance through the education system.

## CHARACTERISTICS OF PROFESSIONAL AND TECHNICAL NURSES OF THE FUTURE AND THEIR EDUCATIONAL PROGRAMS

The characteristics of professional and technical nurses are basic descriptors of the graduates of nursing programs of the future. These characteristics follow from the nursing needs of patients and the health care environment of the year 2000.

## PROFESSIONAL NURSES

### Education

Educational programs to prepare professional nurses of the future will be different than those of today. They will consist of liberal education and nursing education components. Changing health care needs, an increased knowledge base, and the impact of technology will stimulate the change in these educational programs. Professional nurses of the future will be graduates of baccalaureate or higher degree programs with a major in nursing.

### Knowledge

The graduates of professional nursing programs of the future will have an understanding and appreciation of various disciplines, a broad perspective which will be achieved through study of multiple content areas. The knowledge base of the professional nurse will include the ability to think logically, analyze critically, and communicate effectively. Professional nurses' scientific background will provide a distinction between observation and inference in scientific investigation. As liberally educated individuals, professional nurses will understand the influence of personal and social values on human behavior.

Nursing knowledge which incorporates all perspectives of nursing science as well as other disciplines will include theory, methods, processes and ways of knowing and understanding, analysis and study of human events and issues that are of importance to nursing. Professional nurses will integrate knowledge from liberal education and nursing and apply this knowledge in client situations.

## TECHNICAL NURSES

### Education

Educational programs to prepare technical nurses of the future will be different than those of today. They will consist of general education courses and natural and behavioral sciences which support the nursing component of the program. Changing client needs, increased knowledge base, and the impact of technology will stimulate the change in the educational programs. Technical nurses of the future will be graduates of associate degree programs in nursing.

## Knowledge

The graduates of technical nursing programs of the future will have an understanding of the common effects of attitudes, beliefs and values of health behavior. The knowledge base of technical nurses will be used for understanding patients' problems from biological, social, and psychological perspectives. The knowledge base of technical nurses will emphasize facts, concepts, and principles, demonstrated relationships and verified observations. Nursing content for technical nurses will include a well-defined body of established nursing skills and knowledge which is applied in a problem-solving way as technical nurses care for individuals and their families experiencing usual, well-defined problems.

## Practice: Skills, Values, Accountability

Professional nurses will assume primary responsibility for assisting individuals, families, and groups to attain their maximum health potential. Professional nurses will be skilled in nursing practice as caregivers, case managers, and problem solvers. These professionals will analyze health care data and diagnose problems for clients in all types of care settings.

Professional nursing practice will include direct care to clients in any setting as well as case management. Encompassed in the direct care of patients, professional nursing practice will include counseling, health education, and the delegation and evaluation of nursing practice. In coordinating care between patients and existing health care services, professional nursing practice will include adjusting plans for the delivery of nursing care and engaging informal support systems and necessary resources. Professional nursing practice will also include nursing administration, education, and research. Professional nurses will make decisions regarding nursing care and develop policies, procedures, and protocols as guidelines for the provision of nursing care.

The Code of Ethics developed by the profession will provide

the framework that guides the decisions and behavior of professional nurses in the clinical situation. Professional nurses will develop systems and ethical standards that govern professional and personal behavior.

Professional nurses will be accountable for all aspects of nursing care and evaluating the outcomes of care delivered. Professional nurses will be directly accountable and responsible for the patient for the quality of nursing care delivered.

## Practice: Skills, Values, Accountability

Technical nurses will be caregivers and participants in developing the plan of care for patients with well-defined health or illness problems.

Technical nurses will be responsible for organizing the individualized care of patients, prioritizing client needs effectively, and implementing care efficiently. Coordination and direction of nursing care will be facilitated through the use of policies, procedures and protocols developed by professional nursing. Technical nursing practice will include providing patient care in a structured environment, implementation of the teaching plan, management of an individual plan of care, and data collection for the evaluation of nursing care. Technical nurses make decisions about the care of individual clients by applying tested criteria and norms.

The Code of Ethics developed by the nursing profession will guide the actions of technical nurses in the clinical setting.

Technical nurses will be accountable for their own actions in the care of patients within the total context of the nursing plan of care using protocols or standards developed by professional nurses. Technical nurses will be responsible and accountable to the patient for nursing care delivered.

## BIBLIOGRAPHY

American Nurses' Association. (1981). *Educational preparation for nursing. A source book.* Kansas City, ANA Publication No. NE-105M 4/81.
American Organization of Nurse Executives Staff. (1986, July/August).

Maine passes model legislation on educational requirements. *The Nurse Executive*, 9–10.

Council of Associate Degree Programs. (1978). *Competencies of the associate degree nurse on entry into practice.* New York: National League for Nursing. No. 23-1731.

Council of Baccalaureate and Higher Degree Programs. (1979). *Characteristics of baccalaureate education in nursing.* New York: National League for Nursing.

Hanner, M. B. (1985). Associate and bachelor's degree preparation for future clinical practice in home health care. *Journal, NYSNA, 16*(4), 31–37.

Johnson, D. E. (1966). Competence in practice: technical and professional. *Nursing Outlook, 14*, 30–33.

Midwest Alliance in Nursing. (1985). Associate Degree Nursing: Facilitating competency development, defining and differentiating nursing competencies. Unpublished report. Dr. P. Primm, Project Director.

New York State Nurses Association. (1978). *Report of the task force on behavioral outcomes of nursing education programs.* Unpublished by the council of nursing education. Albany.

North Dakota Board of Nursing. 1986. *Administrative rules, article 54-03.1, requirements for nursing education program.* Bismark, ND: Author.

Stevens, B.J. (1985). Does the 1985 nursing education proposal make economic sense? *Nursing Outlook, 33*, 124–127.

Styles, M.M. (1985, July). *The future market place, regulation of health care providers and education of nurses.* Paper presented at the conference on nursing in the 21st century sponsored by AACN, AONE, Aspen, CO.

Texas Nurses' Association. (1983). *Directions for nursing education in Texas 1983–1995: An operational plan.* Unpublished report of the council on education. Austin, TX.

The Professional Preparation Project. (1986). *Seven liberal outcomes of professional study.* Ann Arbor, MI: University of Michigan.

Vermont Nurses' Association. (1985). *Vermont registered nurse, 51*(4).

Wisconsin Task Force. (1982). *Competencies of two levels of nurses.* Madison, WI: University of Wisconsin-Madison.

# 2
# Demographics
# of RN/Baccalaureate
# Education Programs

## PROGRAMS AND INSTITUTIONS

An understanding of the overall institutional context in which RN/ BSN education exists is important when discussing this movement. Bachelor's degree programs in nursing are offered in 606 senior colleges and universities. About one third ($n$ = 203, 34%) of these schools also offer the master's degree in nursing; 7% ($n$ = 43), the doctoral degree in nursing; and 14% ($n$ = 85), the associate degree in nursing.

Of the colleges/universities that offer the BSN, about half classify themselves as under public sponsorship and half as under private sponsorship. Table 2.1 displays the distribution of baccalaureate programs in nursing by the kind of institution in which they are located, as defined by the Carnegie classification of institutions of higher education (Carnegie Foundation, 1987; see Table 2.2).

Table 2.1 shows that BSN programs are offered in more than two thirds of doctorate-granting institutions and comprehensive universities and colleges. Fewer liberal arts colleges offer a BSN. Those programs offered in specialized institutions may be clustered with medical schools or other schools of the health professions. They may also be single-purpose schools of nursing.

About half of the nursing units are schools within the college/ university, and half are departments or divisions within a school or

**TABLE 2.1. Schools of Nursing in the Four-Year Higher Education Sector by Carnegie Classification (N = 606)**

| Institution | Total No. Schools in U.S. | Schools of Nursing | % Schools of Nursing of Total | % Schools of Nursing |
|---|---|---|---|---|
| Doctorate-granting institutions | 173 | 111 | 64 | 18 |
| Research universities I | 52 | 42 | 81 | 7 |
| Research universities II | 40 | 14 | 35 | 2 |
| Doctorate-granting universities I | 53 | 26 | 49 | 4 |
| Doctorate-granting universities II | 58 | 29 | 50 | 5 |
| Comprehensive universities and colleges | 456 | 322 | 71 | 53 |
| I | 323 | 244 | 76 | 40 |
| II | 133 | 78 | 59 | 13 |
| Liberal arts colleges | 721 | 138 | 19 | 23 |
| I | 146 | 19 | 13 | 3 |
| II | 575 | 119 | 21 | 20 |
| Specialized institutions | 424 | 33 | 8 | 5 |

Carnegie Foundation for the Advancement of Teaching, *A Classification of Institutions of Higher Education*, The Foundation, Princeton, NJ, 1987.

college. Fifteen percent of the programs may be classified as being administratively part of an academic health center, defined as an administrative unit that includes a school of medicine, a teaching hospital, and at least one additional health education program. An

**Table 2.2. Carnegie Classifications**

Research universities I
  These institutions offer a full range of baccalaureate programs, are committed to graduate education through the
  doctoral degree, and give high priority to research. They
  receive annually at least $33.5 million in federal support
  and award at least 50 PhD degrees each year.
Research universities II
  These institutions offer a full range of baccalaureate programs, are committed to graduate education through the
  doctoral degree, and give high priority to research. They
  received annually between $12.5 million and $33.5 million
  in federal support for research and development and award
  at least 50 PhD degrees each year.
Doctorate-granting universities I
  In addition to offering a full range of baccalaureate programs,
  the mission of these institutions includes a commitment to
  graduate education through the doctoral degree. They
  award at least 40 PhD degrees annually in five or more
  academic disciplines.
Doctorate-granting universities II
  In addition to offering a full range of baccalaureate programs,
  the mission of these institutions includes a commitment to
  graduate education through the doctoral degree. They
  award annually 20 or more PhD degrees in at least one
  discipline or 100 or more PhD degrees in three or more
  disciplines.
Comprehensive universities and colleges I
  These institutions offer baccalaureate programs and, with few
  exceptions, graduate education through the master's degree.
  More than half of their baccalaureate degrees are awarded
  in two or more occupational or professional disciplines,
  such as engineering or business administration. All of the
  institutions in this group enroll at least 2,500 students.
Comprehensive universities and colleges II
  These institutions award more than half of their baccalaureate
  degrees in two or more occupational or professional disciplines, such as engineering or business administration, and

**Table 2.2.  (Continued)**

---

many also offer graduate education through the master's degree. All of the colleges and universities in this group enroll between 1,500 and 2,500 students.

Liberal arts colleges I
  These highly selective institutions are primarily undergraduate colleges that award more than half of their baccalaureate degrees in arts and science fields.
Liberal arts colleges II
  These institutions are primarily undergraduate colleges that are less selective and award more than half of their degrees in liberal arts fields. This category also includes a group of colleges that award fewer than half of their degrees in liberal arts fields but, with fewer than 1,500 students, are too small to be considered comprehensive.
Professional schools and other specialized institutions
  These institutions offer degrees ranging from the bachelor's to the doctorate. At least 50% of the degrees awarded by these institutions are in a single specialized field. Specialized institutions include theological seminaries, medical schools; schools of law, schools of business management, and schools of arts, music and design.

---

*Source.* The Carnegie Foundation for the Advancement of Teaching A Classification of Institutions of Higher Education, The Foundation, Princeton, N.J., 1987.

academic health center may be part of a university or may be a freestanding institution.

Figure 2.1 shows the distribution of BSN programs by region. Fourteen percent of the programs are located in rural areas, 34% in small cities (25,000–100,000 population), 43% in metropolitan areas, and 9% in inner cities. In all, the nursing education enterprise in 4-year colleges and universities enrolled 149,864 students in 1986 (81,602 BSN, 46,355 RN/BSN, 19,958 MSN, and 1,949 doctoral students) and employed 9,184 faculty (NLN, 1988).

Terminology to describe baccalaureate education for RNs is confusing. Hart and Sharp (1986) describe the plethora of terms that refer to selectivity of admission, to the tightness of the articulation

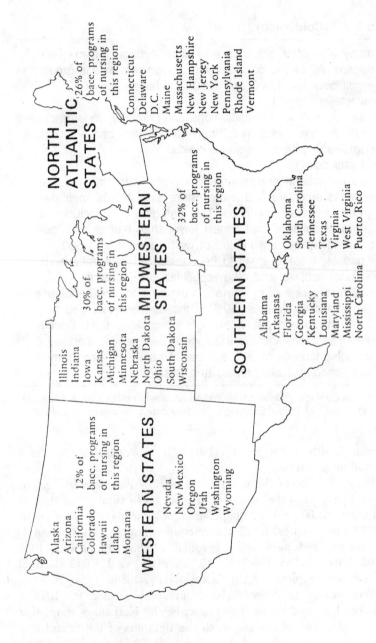

**NORTH ATLANTIC STATES**

26% of bacc. programs of nursing in this region

Connecticut
Delaware
D.C.
Maine
Massachusetts
New Hampshire
New Jersey
New York
Pennsylvania
Rhode Island
Vermont

**MIDWESTERN STATES**

30% of bacc. programs of nursing in this region

Illinois
Indiana
Iowa
Kansas
Michigan
Minnesota
Nebraska
North Dakota
Ohio
South Dakota
Wisconsin

**WESTERN STATES**

12% of bacc. programs of nursing in this region

Alaska
Arizona
California
Colorado
Hawaii
Idaho
Montana
Nevada
New Mexico
Oregon
Utah
Washington
Wyoming

**SOUTHERN STATES**

32% of bacc. programs of nursing in this region

Alabama
Arkansas
Florida
Georgia
Kentucky
Louisiana
Maryland
Mississippi
North Carolina
Oklahoma
South Carolina
Tennessee
Texas
Virginia
West Virginia
Puerto Rico

**Figure 2.1** Concentration of BSN programs by region

with previous nursing/preparation and to the options for entry to and exit from the program. None of this terminology has been well standardized.

Because much of the literature debates whether it is possible to educate RN students adequately in generic programs and why it is important to create separate tracks for these students, we chose to focus on this issue in the classification of programs. Basically, the options are twofold: to integrate RNs into the generic program and to create a separate program for them, frequently in institutions that do not offer generic baccalaureate education. A program designed especially for RNs admitted with junior standing may be called an upper 2; if it is articulated with an associate degree program, it may be called a 2 + 2; both of these patterns have been called second-step programs. Although some second-step programs began in the late 1960s, most were not operating until the mid-1970s.

As can be seen in Table 2.3, the most common pattern was to integrate RNs directly into the generic program (46% of all programs). Most other schools have designed a separate track or program for RNs, but in many instances they intermix generic students and RNs for some nursing coursework and/or clinical experiences (30% of programs). In about one quarter of the institutions, the only baccalaureate-level offering in nursing is the RN completion program. It must be noted as well that only a tiny minority of schools do not admit RNs at all (3% of programs); thus, the BSN is more available for RNs than it is for generic students.

Again, using the Carnegie classification of institutions of higher education, Table 2.4 shows that institutions offering RN completion programs span all of the institutional classifications, but such programs are more likely to be located in liberal arts colleges (II) and in comprehensive universities and colleges than are programs in which RNs are to some degree integrated with an ongoing generic nursing program. The RN completion program pattern is concentrated in schools and departments of nursing offering undergraduate education only. About one third of schools of nursing offer the master's degree, whereas only 10% of those offering RN completion programs offer a master's. Eight percent of U.S. schools of nursing offer the doctoral degree, but only 3% of those with RN completion

**TABLE 2.3. Types of Baccalaureate Programs for RNs Offered by Schools[a]**

| Type of program | No. | % |
|---|---|---|
| Generic program with RN students integrated directly into the generic program | 211 | 45.8 |
| Generic program where RN students are admitted into a *separate* baccalaureate completion program/track but take some nursing coursework and/or clinical experiences with generic students | 138 | 29.9 |
| Generic program and a *separate* baccalaureate completion program/track where RN students *do not* take any coursework with generic students | 21 | 4.6 |
| No generic program; have only an RN baccalaureate completion program | 109 | 23.6 |
| RN external degree baccalaureate completion program[b] | 3 | 0.7 |

[a]Some schools offer two types of programs, frequently in transition from one type to another.
[b]External degree is defined as a degree awarded by transcript evaluation or academically acceptable cognitive and performance examinations. Students can earn the entire degree through examination; however, many students combine college coursework and examination.

programs offer the doctoral degree. In the schools that offer an ADN in addition to the bachelor's degree (14%), not surprisingly, the RN completion program is the most common pattern of RN/BSN education. Within regions, there are different distributions of program types, (see Table 2.5).

Table 2.6 presents enrollment statistics for all respondent BSN programs for the past several years. Although all programs serving RNs have increased dramatically in enrollment, perhaps the biggest increases have occurred in those programs that integrate RNs into generic programs and among part-time students. RN student enrollment has increased considerably during a time when generic stu-

**TABLE 2.4.  Classification of Respondent Institution's Program Type by Carnegie Classification (*n* = 461)**

| Carnegie classification | RNs integrated with generics | | RN completion | |
|---|---|---|---|---|
| | No | % | No. | % |
| Research I | 31 | 9.5 | 4 | 3.0 |
| Research II | 11 | 3.4 | 1 | .7 |
| Doctorate-granting universities I | 21 | 6.4 | 3 | 2.2 |
| Doctorate-granting universities II | 22 | 6.7 | 5 | 3.7 |
| Comprehensive universities and colleges | | | | |
| I | 123 | 37.6 | 57 | 42.5 |
| II | 33 | 10.1 | 19 | 14.2 |
| Liberal arts colleges | | | | |
| I | 8 | 2.4 | 3 | 2.2 |
| II | 55 | 16.8 | 36 | 26.9 |
| Specialized institutions | 17 | 5.2 | 3 | 2.2 |
| Not classifiable | 6 | 1.8 | 3 | 2.2 |

**TABLE 2.5.  Regional Distribution of Program Types**

| Program types | Northeast | Midwest | South | West |
|---|---|---|---|---|
| RN students in generic programs | 20% | 13% | 28% | 19% |
| RNs somewhat integrated with generics | 26% | 40% | 34% | 19% |
| RNs separate from generics | 16% | 21% | 20% | 17% |
| RN completion program (no generic) | 39% | 26% | 19% | 46% |

**TABLE 2.6. Baccalaureate Student Enrollment by Type of Program**

| Type of BSN program | Fall 1984 | | Fall 1985 | | Fall 1986 | | % Change 1984–86 |
|---|---|---|---|---|---|---|---|
| | No. of schools | No. of students | No. of schools | No. of students | No. of schools | No. of students | |
| Generic students | | | | | | | |
| FT | 314 | 70,579 | 324 | 65,492 | 336 | 58,581 | 17.0 |
| PT | 314 | 8952 | 324 | 8851 | 336 | 8933 | 0.2 |
| COM | 314 | 79,531 | 324 | 74,343 | 336 | 67,514 | 15.1 |
| RNs integrated into generic program | | | | | | | |
| FT | 180 | 1684 | 187 | 1532 | 207 | 1749 | 3.9 |
| PT | 180 | 5246 | 187 | 5670 | 207 | 6673 | 27.2 |
| COM | 180 | 6930 | 187 | 7202 | 207 | 8422 | 21.5 |
| RNs in separate program but have some courses with generic | | | | | | | |
| FT | 87 | 2008 | 98 | 1804 | 106 | 2048 | 2.0 |
| PT | 87 | 4127 | 98 | 4736 | 106 | 4996 | 21.1 |
| COM | 87 | 6135 | 98 | 6540 | 106 | 7044 | 14.8 |

| | | | | | | | |
|---|---|---|---|---|---|---|---|
| **RNs in separate program from generic** | | | | | | | |
| FT | 26 | 1222 | 26 | 1163 | 31 | 1306 | 6.9 |
| PT | 26 | 2563 | 26 | 3128 | 31 | 3134 | 22.3 |
| COM | 26 | 3785 | 26 | 4291 | 31 | 4440 | 17.3 |
| **RN-only program** | | | | | | | |
| FT | 89 | 1592 | 94 | 1722 | 99 | 1856 | 16.6 |
| PT | 89 | 7975 | 94 | 8300 | 99 | 8784 | 10.1 |
| COM | 89 | 9567 | 94 | 10,022 | 99 | 10,640 | 11.2 |
| **External degree program** | | | | | | | |
| FT | a | 0 | a | 0 | 3 | 0 | |
| PT | a | 5361 | a | 5552 | 3 | 5272 | 1.7 |
| COM | a | 5361 | a | 5552 | 3 | 5272 | 1.7 |
| **All RN** | | | | | | | |
| FT | 370 | 6506 | 394 | 6221 | 422 | 6959 | 7.0 |
| PT | 370 | 25,272 | 394 | 27,386 | 422 | 28,859 | 14.2 |
| COM | 370 | 31,778 | 394 | 33,607 | 422 | 35,818 | 12.7 |
| **Generic and RN, total BSN** | | | | | | | |
| FT | 409 | 77,085 | 422 | 71,713 | 441 | 65,540 | 5.0 |
| PT | 409 | 34,224 | 422 | 36,237 | 441 | 37,792 | 10.4 |
| COM | 409 | 111,309 | 422 | 107,950 | 441 | 103,332 | 7.2 |

aFewer than 3 schools reporting.
FT, full-time; PT, part-time; COM, combined full-time and part-time.

dent enrollment declined 15%. The distribution of RN enrollment in fall 1986 in the various program types is shown in Table 2.7.

Two thirds of deans reported that their RN/BSN programs would be expanding; those in which RN students are integrated with or parallel with generic students were more likely to expect expansion (61–78%) than RN completion programs (49% expected to expand) ($\chi^2[3, n = 414] = 11.22, p = .011$). It is important to note that of the 461 respondent institutions, 45 had established their programs for RNs between 1984 and 1987.

Eighty-two percent of program heads reported their programs were NLN-accredited, and nearly 10% said that their programs were new and therefore not yet eligible for voluntary accreditation. An important fact to remember is that all states require that programs preparing students for initial licensure be accredited by the state board of nursing (or another state-level board). This may not be the case for programs in which students are RNs since they are already licensed. Twenty-eight percent of programs report that their RN/BSN programs are under the jurisdiction of the board of nurs-

**TABLE 2.7. Distribution of RN Enrollment in Fall 1986**

| Program types | % Total RN/BSN enrollment ($n = 461$) |
|---|---|
| RNs integrated into the generic program | 24 |
| RNs enrolled in separate baccalaureate completion program/track but take some courses with generics | 20 |
| RNs enrolled in separate baccalaureate completion program/track and do not take courses with generics | 12 |
| RN program only (do not have generic program) | 36 |
| RNs enrolled in external degree baccalaureate completion program | 9 |

ing. A survey of state boards of nursing found that in only 12 states and the District of Columbia do the boards of nursing approve RN completion/advanced placement programs. The states are Delaware, Georgia, Idaho, Iowa, Nevada, New Jersey, North Dakota, Oregon, Tennessee, Texas, Vermont, and Wyoming.

All programs under the jurisdiction of the board of nursing were reported to be fully or conditionally approved or were new programs. Under such a policy, an average of 70% of the eligible students were reported to take the exam prior to completion of the BSN, and of those, 88% passed it. An average of 40% of those students successfully passing the licensure exam returned to the BSN program as part-time students. Nearly one third did not return to the program the following enrollment period.

In California, until 1987, all nursing programs were required to include content that would enable students to take the licensing examination by the time they had completed 36 months in the program. This regulation was rescinded in 1987, and it is now up to the school whether or not it wants to follow this pattern.

## FACULTY AND STUDENTS

The "average" program reported having 16 full-time and 5 part-time faculty, as well as 28 adjunct faculty and preceptors. Forty percent of the faculty teaching on the baccalaureate level were tenured. Interestingly, 43% of schools reported that they have both tenure- and nontenure-track appointments; only 10% report having no tenure track at all. Having no tenure track is more common at 4-year colleges (16%) than at universities (6%) ($\chi^2[2, n = 434] = 14.05, p < .001$).

One fifth of the faculty teaching in baccalaureate programs were doctorally prepared, and 75% held the master's as their terminal degree. About 40% of those faculty established their clinical specialty as medical-surgical/adult health, 16% as community health, 15% as psychiatric/mental health, 13% as ob-gyn/women's health, 12% as pediatrics, and 5% as other.

Student respondents were 96% female and 9% minority. Average age was 36 years, ranging from 20 to 62. Fifty-nine percent were married, and 57% had children. Seven percent had previously earned a bachelor's degree in another field. Generic students as a group include slightly higher percentages of males (6%) and of minorities (17%). Non-Caucasian RN students were significantly more likely to be represented in programs located in inner cities (22% of RN students) than in programs located in rural areas (6%), metropolitan areas (12%), or small cities (6%) [$F$ (3,355) = 10.11, $p$ <.001].

## ADEQUACY OF RESOURCES

Competition for funds is an ongoing concern in higher education. Most deans felt that their baccalaureate programs in nursing were being given funds equivalent to other same-size programs in their institutions (60%) or were given higher priority for funds (30%), although 27% felt their budgets were still inadequate. Although 8% of deans felt that their baccalaureate programs were given low priority, 5% believed that their programs were very inadequately funded, and 19% reported that their budgets were lower for 1986–87 than for 1985–86, the more usual picture was of adequate budgets (73%) and budgets that were higher (53%) or at the same level (22%) than the previous year. Interestingly, 80% of those who thought their schools received low priority for funds within the institution were in universities, and 20% were in 4-year colleges ($\chi^2[2, n = 429] = 10.500, p$ <.005). A further comparison shows that 92% of those not in academic health centers felt that their program received high priority for funding, whereas those in academic health centers were more likely to feel that their funds were equivalent, with only 8% believing that their programs received high priority ($\chi^2[2, n = 432] = 9.15, p$ <.010).

Of those schools that have both generic and RN programs, most (79%) reported that both programs received the same budget priority. Eighteen percent reported giving higher priority to their generic programs, and 3% reported higher priority for their RN programs.

Table 2.8 provides data about the deans' perceived adequacy of particular kinds of resources. There appear to be few differences

**TABLE 2.8. Deans' Perceptions of Adequacy of Specific Resources for Baccalaureate Education ($n = 461$)**

| Resources | RN students | | | Generic students | | |
|---|---|---|---|---|---|---|
| | No. | Mean[a] | S.D. | No. | Mean[a] | S.D. |
| Audiovisual equipment | 406 | 4.72 | 1.27 | 339 | 4.75 | 1.29 |
| Library collection in nursing | 404 | 4.66 | 1.28 | 337 | 4.67 | 1.32 |
| Administrative/faculty office space | 406 | 4.56 | 1.47 | 339 | 4.66 | 1.48 |
| Classroom space | 404 | 4.51 | 1.49 | 340 | 4.57 | 1.50 |
| Computer services/computer time | 400 | 4.42 | 1.43 | 337 | 4.50 | 1.43 |
| Funding for BSN program(s) | 397 | 4.22 | 1.41 | 340 | 4.34 | 1.34 |
| Meeting/conference room space | 406 | 4.20 | 1.55 | 341 | 4.25 | 1.57 |
| Funding for academic advisement | 308 | 4.17 | 1.51 | 260 | 4.18 | 1.50 |
| Funding for full-time faculty salaries | 399 | 4.11 | 1.51 | 341 | 4.09 | 1.52 |
| Secretarial support services | 403 | 4.06 | 1.50 | 341 | 4.11 | 1.51 |
| Funding for part-time faculty salaries | 368 | 3.96 | 1.53 | 317 | 3.99 | 1.46 |
| Student space (study areas, etc.) | 392 | 3.85 | 1.65 | 334 | 3.99 | 1.61 |
| Program development | 388 | 3.76 | 1.49 | 324 | 3.73 | 1.46 |
| Consultation | 375 | 3.62 | 1.52 | 314 | 3.60 | 1.49 |

(continued)

**TABLE 2.8.  (Continued)**

| Resources | RN students | | | Generic students | | |
|---|---|---|---|---|---|---|
| | No. | Mean[a] | S.D. | No. | Mean[a] | S.D. |
| Funding for faculty development | 404 | 3.57 | 1.57 | 335 | 3.59 | 1.55 |
| Funding for disadvantaged student ongoing advisement | 244 | 3.41 | 1.62 | 229 | 3.40 | 1.60 |
| Funding for student recruitment | 350 | 3.39 | 1.58 | 301 | 3.45 | 1.59 |
| Funding for clinical preceptors | 145 | 3.10 | 1.85 | 123 | 3.16 | 1.83 |
| Renovation | 327 | 3.08 | 1.59 | 284 | 3.11 | 1.66 |
| Funding for faculty research | 366 | 2.93 | 1.54 | 314 | 3.01 | 1.54 |

[a]1, very inadequate; 2, moderately inadequate; 3, slightly inadequate; 4, slightly adequate; 5, moderately adequate; 6, very adequate.

between programs for RN students and those for generics. The results support findings from more global studies about adequacy of support (Gunne, 1985). Besides money for renovation, funding for faculty research was clearly perceived to be the most inadequately funded area. Schools in academic health centers and those with NLN accreditation report more adequate funding than do others.

On the average, this population of schools reports that half of their budgets come from tuition and/or state funds. The amount from tuition was reported as having increased, but on the average, money from federal support grants, private funds, and state funds did not change.

## SUMMARY

As pointed out in Chapter 1, the present phenomenon of large numbers of RN students earning the bachelor's degree is an additional phase in the transition of nursing to higher levels of university-based education. The RN Baccalaureate Nursing Data Project on which this book is based explored the system of education in which RNs are enrolled, beginning with this chapter describing the demographics of RN/BSN education.

One particular trend identified in the demographic data raises an important issue. The few states that mandate that students have the opportunity to take the RN licensing exam prior to graduation from the baccalaureate program may be unwittingly adding to the costs to be incurred by the educational system. In the RN Baccalaureate Nursing Data Project approximately one third of students in these programs did not re-enroll in their bachelor's degree program the semester after taking the RN exam. It is highly likely that at some point these students will be seeking the opportunity to complete the bachelor's degree. However, what is not equally likely is that students who leave without the bachelor's degree and successfully complete the RN licensing exam will remain at the site of initial education. These students will request accommodation by the educational system later and perhaps require costs in excess of those that might have been incurred had the baccalaureate been completed during initial education.

## REFERENCES

American Council on Education. (1986). *1986–87 fact book on higher education*. New York: Macmillan.

Carnegie Foundation for the Advancement of Teaching. (1987). *A classification of institutions of higher education*. Princeton, NJ: Author.

Gunne, G. M. (1985). The fiscal status of nursing education programs in the United States. *Journal of Professional Nursing, 1,* 336–347.

Hart, S. E., & Sharp, T. G. (1986). Mobility programs for students and faculty. In National League for Nursing (Ed.), *Looking beyond the entry for nursing*. New York: Author.

National League for Nursing. (1988). *Nursing data review, 1987*. New York: Author.

# 3

# Access and Motivation

Access to BSN education has been a concern for RNs for some time, as the system of nursing education has shifted into a model quite different in its assumptions and practices from that of diploma education. The history of articulation and transfer between 2-year and 4-year institutions in higher education has never been a well-defined pathway. Much has been left to the discretion of individual institutions both in structuring the education to facilitate transfer (2-year institutions) and in fitting credits into a bachelor's degree program (4-year institutions).

Access must be addressed from several perspectives: (1) geographic access, (2) time access, (3) financial access, (4) psychological access, and (5) ability to recoup previous investment in education. All of these questions, with the possible exception of the last, are concerns of all adult learners, and one would presume that these conditions interact with motivation to attain the BSN. That is, motivation would be stimulated in part by ease of access, and policies to improve access are likely to be adopted in response to strong demand for the degree from RN students. This strong demand may in turn be motivated by signals from the environment about qualifications for career development and by interest in self-development. All of these facets of access are jointly defined by both the potential student and the educational institution.

*Geographic access* is simply distance and ease of travel from residence or site of work to site of instruction. It is assumed that most adult learners will not relocate, and because most continue to be employed, they would like instruction to be located as close as possible to their homes or places of work. Institutions have relaxed residency requirements and made instruction available at off-campus or outreach sites and sometimes at places of employment.

*Time access* involves (1) structuring the curriculum so that it can be completed in small blocks at a time and (2) offering instruction at times when people are not working. *Financial access* involves individuals' abilities to pay for their education and their access to student financial assistance commonly available to other students. It requires balancing financial commitments incurred as an adult with investment in one's education.

*Psychological access* seems to involve two factors. One is the self-redefinition necessary to return to student status, bolstered by the motivation behind such an important decision. This factor is well defined in adult education literature; it includes (1) resolving problems of insecurity about the ability to succeed, the decision to return, and family and work responsibilities and (2) dealing with the fear that skills, knowledge, and abilities acquired as a younger learner may no longer be appropriate, especially in light of one's current image of oneself as an autonomous person with established ways of learning (Callin, 1983). The second factor in psychological access involves sufficient orientation to institutions of higher education to know how to access information, solve problems, and negotiate with the institution for admission and placement. In fact, lack of proficiency in these skills can be interpreted by RNs or other adult learners as psychological rejection by the institution.

An enormous amount of effort has been invested, particularly in nursing, in the issue of transfer of credit and validation of previous learning, the aspect of access one might call the *ability to recoup previous investment in education*. It has definitely been perceived as a barrier to access. It is perhaps more clearly seen as a clash between the culture and traditional practices of colleges and universities, which have been established to safeguard quality, and the experiential orientation of work on which apprenticeship education is based.

The nursing literature describes issues of psychological and previous-investment access as experienced by RN students: the fear that competence as a nurse will be challenged at every turn and that perhaps one will no longer be labeled a professional; the need to reject, to a certain degree, some prior values, norms, and standards in order to enter into a new nursing culture; the shock described by one student at learning how little college credit she received for 3 years of diploma education (Brainerd, 1983; Williams, 1984).

These concerns about access/motivation and the price one is paying for the experience and the degree can affect the student's and faculty's educational experience throughout the BSN program. Some have charged that colleges and universities have focused many of their services—including career development, counseling programs, and support services—too exclusively on needs of traditional-age students (Griff, 1987). Indeed, the notion of student retention and satisfaction as indicators of institutional effectiveness is gaining credence in larger discussions of college and university performance (Astin, Korn, & Green, 1987).

Concerns about access are, of course, tangled with students' pressures and motivations in pursuing the baccalaureate. In one school of nursing, Arlton (1983) found that the two reasons most frequently cited by RN students for obtaining the BSN were (1) perceived pressure by the profession to become eligible for promotion and supervising positions and (2) the need to prepare for graduate education. Fulfilling a need to learn and to know was least frequently cited (Arlton, 1983). Indeed, the organized nursing profession is moving vigorously toward clear differentiation between the professional and technical practice of nursing. Following is the American Nurses' Association's (1987) position on the scope of nursing practice.

### Differences Between the Professional and Technical Practice of Nursing

The depth and breadth to which the individual nurse engages in the total scope of the clinical practice of nursing are defined by the knowledge base of the nurse, the role of the nurse, and the nature of the client population within a practice environment. In the future, these same characteristics will differentiate the professional and technical practice of nursing.

Knowledge Base of the Nurse

Differences between the knowledge base for professional and technical nursing practice are both quantitative and qualitative. Education for professional practice is provided within baccalaureate or higher degree programs with a major in nursing. Set within the framework of liberal education, these programs provide for the study of nursing theory within the context of related scientific, behavioral, and humanistic disciplines. Graduates of professional programs have the knowledge base requisite for additional formal education in specialized clinical practice, nursing research, nursing administation, and nursing education.

Graduates of professional programs are prepared to engage in the full scope of the clinical practice of nursing. They must be educated to understand the various modes of nursing inquiry and the principles of scientific investigation and must be able to synthesize relevant information and make clinical inferences. They must know how to project patient outcomes, establish nursing plans of care to achieve those outcomes, and evaluate the patient's response to nursing intervention. They must apply nursing theory to the assessment, diagnosis, treatment, and evaluation of human responses to health and illness in both the individual clinical situation and the broader community setting.

Education for the technical practice of nursing is provided in community colleges or other institutions of higher education qualified to offer the associate degree in nursing. Set within the framework of general education, these programs provide for the study of nursing within the context of the applied sciences. Clinical content is empirical in nature and focuses on skills, facts, demonstrated relationships, and experientially verified observations.

Graduates of associate degree programs are prepared to engage in the technical aspects of the clinical practice of nursing. They must have the knowledge base to apply a circumscribed body of established nursing principles and skills. They must be educated to understand patient problems from a biological, social, and psychological perspective, and to use a problem-solving approach to the health care of individuals and their families in a variety of organized nursing service settings.

In addition, the recent American Hospital Association (AHA, 1987) data showing nurse executives' desire for more educated staff also provided evidence of the pressures on RNs prepared at the associate degree and diploma levels to increase their education preparation.

The following section reports data about access and motivation obtained from deans of schools of nursing that accept RN students for the BSN and from the senior RN/BSN students themselves.

## SCHOOL PRACTICES THAT AFFECT ACCESS AND MOTIVATION

Recruitment activities, program capacity to accept RNs, and scheduling and sites of classes are institutional decisions that presumably affect access. Table 3.1 presents data on recruitment strategies used by schools, as reported by both the schools and the senior student sample, and their perceived effectiveness. Both schools and students report that one of the most useful strategies, used by about half of the responding schools, is employing a nurse recruiter for the RN nursing program. Both also agreed that the presence of faculty and students working in clinical agencies was very effective in attracting RN students to the program. RN students also saw attendance at continuing education programs offered by the nursing program and contact with the program's alumnae as moderately effective. Some deans reported that their schools regularly make presentations to senior classes of associate degree and diploma nursing schools, and several reported that they had formalized articulation agreements with these programs.

The relatively low use of videotapes, advertisements, and television and radio was consistent with schools' reported practice for recruitment of RN and generic students. Students also report that these methods are very ineffective. Deans reported increasing recruitment for RN students over their previous year's efforts, pointing out that there is competition from other schools for students.

It is interesting to note how few recruitment strategies RN students perceived as being used, perhaps in part because they reflect only on their own experience. In addition, some recruitment activities may be new since these students entered the program. In additional comments, students noted that they were attracted to the school because friends were enrolled, because of its location, and because classes were held at the hospital where they worked.

Eighty-four percent of respondent schools indicated that they do not limit the number of RNs accepted per year. Those that limit enrollment reported lack of faculty resources, budget, and lack of clinical placements as reasons. In 95% of programs there was no waiting list for admission of RNs into the bachelor's degree program. Students verified this statistic; only 3% indicated that they were placed on a waiting list for an average of 6 months before admission into the program. Sixty-one percent of schools reported that they planned to expand their RN programs/tracks within the next 5 years.

Time and geographic access factors are being taken into account by academic institutions to meet the needs of RN students. Sixteen percent of schools reported offering a weekend program; 64%, an evening program; and 56%, a year-round program (including summers). Fourteen percent of senior students reported having used a weekend scheduling option; 66%, an evening program; and 58%, a summer option.

Availability of these options does vary to some extent by geographic area, type of school, and program. For example, weekend programs are more likely to exist in 4-year colleges than in universities ($\chi^2[1, n = 444] = 6.57, p < .010$) and are more common in RN completion programs (82%) than in generic programs in which RNs are placed (35–69%). Weekend programs are also more common in the Midwest (73% of schools) and the Northeast (70% of schools) than in the South (63% of schools) or the West (46% of schools) ($\chi^2[3, n = 449] = 15.10, p < .002$). Such programs are also less likely to be found in schools located in the inner city (48%) than in those in other areas (65–71%). The year-round option is most available in the Midwest (71% of schools) and least available in the West (31% of schools) ($\chi^2[3, n = 449] = 27.46, p < .001$), and more available in private schools (64%) than in schools under public sponsorship (52%) ($\chi^2[2, n = 449] = 6.17, p < .046$).

Geographic access concerns have also been addressed through the use of satellite or outreach programs offered off the main campus of an academic institution: at work sites or many miles away from the academic institution. As might be expected, programs located in rural areas offered significantly more outreach/satellite sites (average, 3.0) than did programs in small cities (average, 2.1) or metropolitan areas (average, 1.9) ($F [3, 165] = 3.28, p = .022$).

**TABLE 3.1. A Comparison of Deans' (n = 461) and RN Students' (n = 742) Perceptions of Effectiveness of RN Recruitment Strategies**

| Strategy | Dean perceptions of effectiveness | | | | Student perceptions of effectiveness | | | |
|---|---|---|---|---|---|---|---|---|
| | No. | Mean[a] | SD | Not used | No. | Mean[a] | SD | Not used |
| Reputation of school/referrals | 415 | 5.41 | .83 | 2 | NA | NA | NA | NA |
| Faculty/students working in clinical agencies | 415 | 5.26 | .89 | 6 | 300 | 4.58 | 1.42 | 428 |
| Nurse recruiter for RN nursing program | 176 | 5.09 | 1.19 | 240 | 229 | 4.32 | 1.61 | 499 |
| Personal letters | 353 | 5.02 | .94 | 64 | 274 | 4.19 | 1.55 | 453 |
| Contact/collaboration with local health care agencies | 409 | 4.95 | .96 | 10 | NA | NA | NA | NA |
| Brochures, pamphlets | 411 | 4.91 | .86 | 8 | 455 | 4.36 | 1.29 | 276 |
| Nursing alumni | 359 | 4.83 | 1.09 | 56 | 265 | 4.85 | 1.32 | 449 |
| Directors of nursing departments | 385 | 4.75 | 1.01 | 30 | NA | NA | NA | NA |
| Collaboration with staff development coordinators at area hospitals | 360 | 4.63 | .98 | 59 | NA | NA | NA | NA |
| Continuing education programs for RNs | 291 | 4.49 | 1.12 | 128 | 139 | 4.32 | 1.60 | 592 |
| Open house | 260 | 4.37 | 1.28 | 162 | 149 | 3.70 | 1.78 | 580 |
| Career fairs | 329 | 4.27 | 1.27 | 94 | 117 | 3.68 | 1.81 | 613 |

| | | | | | | | |
|---|---|---|---|---|---|---|---|
| Magazine/newspaper advertisements | 217 | 4.19 | 1.17 | 203 | 143 | 3.64 | 1.73 | 586 |
| RN refresher courses | 66 | 4.00 | 1.48 | 352 | 57 | 3.37 | 2.03 | 671 |
| Television/radio | 126 | 3.91 | 1.27 | 291 | 85 | 3.38 | 1.89 | 640 |
| Nursing conferences and convention exhibits (ANA, NLN, state) | 238 | 3.90 | 1.29 | 180 | 78 | 3.41 | 1.83 | 652 |
| Videotapes | 116 | 3.84 | 1.35 | 301 | 60 | 2.83 | 1.98 | 669 |
| Nursing journal advertisements | 114 | 3.68 | 1.28 | 300 | 71 | 3.18 | 1.88 | 660 |
| Use of college/university central recruitment office | 358 | 3.65 | 1.56 | 59 | 175 | 3.79 | 1.68 | 554 |

[a]1, very ineffective; 2, slightly ineffective; 3, moderately ineffective; 4, slightly effective; 5, moderately effective; 6, very effective; NA, not on RN student questionnaire.

Indeed, 17% of the students in RN-only programs or in generic programs with no shared courses indicated they had not taken courses on campus, whereas 58% of students from these programs had taken coursework at off-campus sites; 41% of those integrated into generic programs had taken off-campus courses. Programs in which RNs were integrated with generic students were least likely of the program types to use satellite or outreach programs (32%) ($\chi^2[3, n = 423] = 10.59, p < .014$).

Sixty-three schools reported using an average of 2.7 satellite/outreach locations for instruction. These schools also reported that 42% of RN students were currently taking courses at these locations. In addition to these options, independent study and external degree programs were available at several institutions in the country.

## STUDENT DECISIONS/MOTIVATIONS

Original preparation in nursing for the student sample was as follows: 54% associate degree, 46% diploma program, and 8% licensed practical nurse. As has been found in previous surveys, those with associate degrees graduated from their original programs much later (mean, 1979; median, 1981) than did those from diploma programs (mean, 1971; median, 1973). There were distinct geographic differences in the mix of original preparation of RN students: in the Northeast, 53% of RN students obtained their original preparation in diploma schools; in the Midwest, 49%; in the South, 39%; and in the West, 31% ($\chi^2 = [3,742] = 18.48, p = .001$).

Half of the RN students indicated they were aware of the differences between associate degree, diploma, and BSN nursing programs at the time they made their initial decisions to enter nursing. Factors that students said influenced them to choose a nursing career when they entered their original nursing programs and factors that influenced their decisions to choose an associate degree or diploma program may be found in Tables 3.2 and 3.3. The response to factors that influenced these individuals to enter nursing for their original preparation were not unlike those of ge-

**TABLE 3.2. Factors That Influenced RN Students to Choose a Nursing Career (*n* = 742)**

| Factor | No. | % |
|---|---|---|
| Desire to work in the health care field | 552 | 74.4 |
| Opportunity to work closely with people | 484 | 65.2 |
| Availability of jobs in the nursing field | 474 | 63.9 |
| Always wanted to be a nurse | 332 | 44.7 |
| Previous experience in health care agency/field | 273 | 36.8 |
| Diverse positions available in nursing | 258 | 34.8 |
| Reputation of nursing as a professional career | 254 | 34.2 |
| Marketability of nursing skills | 179 | 24.1 |
| Good salary | 164 | 22.1 |
| Flexibility of hours | 135 | 18.2 |
| Opportunity for advancement in nursing positions | 107 | 14.4 |
| Scholarship/financial aid available to study nursing | 64 | 8.6 |

**TABLE 3.3. Factors That Influenced Senior RN/BSN Students to Choose Their Original ADN/Diploma Program (*n* = 742)**

| Factor | No. | % |
|---|---|---|
| Reasonable costs/tuition | 499 | 67.3 |
| Length of program | 462 | 62.3 |
| Convenient location of school | 456 | 61.5 |
| Recommendation of a nurse | 137 | 18.5 |
| Publicity/brochures about program | 131 | 17.7 |
| Recommendation of parents | 125 | 16.8 |
| Recommendation of school counselor | 101 | 13.6 |
| Recommendation of peers | 92 | 12.4 |

neric baccalaureate students. RN students also reported that family influence was strong.

What is startling about the material presented in Table 3.3 is how little sense of investment in education for a professional career RN students appeared to have—programs were chosen because of convenience, length of time to complete, and cost. Today there is evidence in at least one state that the cost of diploma education is very nearly comparable to that of baccalaureate education in the public sector (Table 3.4; Smith, 1986). In addition, a recently completed AACN (1989) study of student costs has shown that the student who chooses associate degree or diploma education as the basic entry preparation will incur greater costs as he or she attempts to complete the bachelor's degree.

Most commonly, students decided to obtain a bachelor's degree some time after completion of their original nursing preparation (56% of respondents). Thirteen percent reported making this decision prior to entering the diploma or associate degree program, 18% while attending the diploma/associate degree program, and 13% some time after completion. Table 3.5 presents information about factors that influenced students' decisions to acquire a bachelor's degree in nursing. Clearly, desire to have a bachelor's degree and the career and educational mobility it affords were important to these students, as was the opportunity for personal and professional growth and development. Again, we see that student decisions were

### TABLE 3.4. Median Tuition for Basic Nursing Education Programs in Maine, 1983–84

| Type of Program | Type of control | |
| --- | --- | --- |
| | Public | Private |
| Associate degree | $3,660 | $10,800 |
| Diploma | — | 5,650 |
| Baccalaureate | 6,257 | 19,600 |

From Smith, D. L. (1986). *Costs of Two Levels of Entry into Nursing Practice to Nursing Students, to Health Care Consumers, and to Institutions, for Nursing Education.* Bangor, ME: Maine State Nurses' Association.

**TABLE 3.5. Factors That Influenced RN Students' Decision to Obtain a Bachelor's Degree in Nursing (*n* = 742)**

| Factor | No. | % |
|---|---|---|
| Greater opportunity for career and educational mobility with a BSN degree | 648 | 87.3 |
| Desire to have a bachelor's degree | 628 | 84.6 |
| More opportunities for personal and professional growth and development | 569 | 76.7 |
| Employment limitations without BSN degree | 486 | 65.5 |
| Desire to pursue an advanced/graduate education | 420 | 56.6 |
| Convenient location of BSN nursing program | 349 | 47.0 |
| Status of having a BSN | 327 | 44.1 |
| Opportunity to work in a nonhospital setting | 317 | 42.7 |
| ANA position paper on entry into practice | 224 | 30.2 |
| Expectation of higher salary with a BSN degree | 212 | 28.6 |
| Time and money already invested in nursing education | 192 | 25.9 |
| Desire for comprehensive liberal arts/scientific background to complement nursing knowledge | 185 | 24.9 |
| Recommendation from nursing service administration to acquire BSN degree (i.e., director of nursing) | 135 | 18.2 |
| Recommendation of faculty member at nursing school | 97 | 13.1 |
| Recommendation from peers to get BSN degree | 95 | 12.8 |
| Recommendation of a nurse | 88 | 11.9 |
| Family expectation to acquire a bachelor's degree | 76 | 10.2 |
| Needed to maintain current nursing position | 76 | 10.2 |
| Recommendation of a school counselor | 15 | 2.0 |

not significantly influenced by school counselors, nurses, or in this instance, nursing faculty.

Pressure from the marketplace was also evident in that nearly two thirds of the students responded to perceived employment limitations without the BSN degree, and a number see status in having a BSN. An extremely interesting finding is the percentage of individuals who returned to acquire the BSN as entrée to the advanced degree program. More than half (56.6%) were motivated by their desire to pursue graduate education.

Few students (15%) applied to more than one baccalaureate nursing program, and those who did indicated they applied to two schools. In choosing a particular baccalaureate program, students noted that acceptance of transfer credits, convenient location, flexibility in scheduling classes/clinical experiences, reasonable costs, and advanced placement opportunities were very important (see Table 3.6). Interestingly, students rated scholarship or grant availability as very unimportant, and more than half indicated that they did not use this factor in their decision making. Students' reported sources of funds to finance their baccalaureate education in nursing

**TABLE 3.6. Mean Degree of Importance for Factors Influencing Selection of Baccalaureate Nursing Program ($n = 742$)**

| Factor | No. | Mean[a] | SD | Did not use |
|---|---|---|---|---|
| Acceptance of transfer credits | 692 | 5.24 | 1.35 | 41 |
| Convenient location | 713 | 5.08 | 1.46 | 16 |
| Flexible schedule of classes/clinical | 656 | 5.02 | 1.42 | 66 |
| Reputation of school | 696 | 4.69 | 1.41 | 31 |
| Reasonable costs/tuition | 705 | 4.61 | 1.53 | 29 |
| Advanced placement opportunities | 545 | 4.42 | 1.76 | 182 |
| Congruence of nursing program with personal philosophy of nursing | 673 | 4.13 | 1.58 | 56 |
| Courses offered off-campus | 385 | 3.67 | 2.19 | 340 |
| Recommendation(s) of family, nurse peers, school and/or counselor | 536 | 3.47 | 1.72 | 189 |
| Scholarship or grant availability | 328 | 3.06 | 2.01 | 403 |
| Day-care facilities offered | 196 | 1.65 | 1.51 | 528 |

[a]1, very unimportant; 2, moderately unimportant; 3, slightly unimportant; 4, slightly important; 5, moderately important; 6, very important

**TABLE 3.7. Student Sources of Educational Financing (N=742)**

| Funding sources | Mean % of students |
|---|---|
| Personal earnings from employment | 53 |
| Employer tuition reimbursement plan | 40 |
| Personal savings | 33 |
| Scholarship/grants | 20 |
| Loans | 16 |
| Spouse | 14 |
| Parents | 7 |

and the adequacy of their financial situations while attending the BSN program are shown in Table 3.7.

Virtually all of these students were currently licensed as RNs, and 87% were currently employed as RNs, working an average of 32 hours per week. Two percent were employed in non-nursing positions, and 8% reported being unemployed. Their earnings and savings, as well as funds from employer tuition reimbursement plans, were clearly major ways in which they financed their education. These RN students' assessment of their financial situation (Table 3.8) was slightly more positive than that reported by generic students, 35% of whom felt that their financial situation during the baccalaureate program was minimal or inadequate (Cassells, Redman, & Jackson, 1986).

**TABLE 3.8. RN Students' Perception of Adequacy of Financial Situation**

| Assessment | % Students ($n$ = 379) |
|---|---|
| Very inadequate | 7 |
| Moderately inadequate | 11 |
| Slightly inadequate | 13 |
| Slightly adequate | 17 |
| Moderately adequate | 33 |
| Very adequate | 19 |

## SUMMARY

Factors related to access and motivation RN students experience when returning to school to obtain the BSN are important not only to these individuals in building their careers but also to the profession and the public in making available needed bachelor's degree nurses. Senior colleges and universities are responding to the need for creative and accessible options for the RN to achieve the BSN degree. The evidence to support this finding is clear: Present senior students in RN/BSN programs reported few delays in obtaining admission to programs; students are using the satellite/outreach locations; and evening, weekend, and year-round instruction opportunities are widely available.

Many of the students returned to school because they felt market pressures or because they identified long-range goals, such as advanced-degree education, that require the bachelor's degree. Many of the students identified a different perspective when choosing their initial preparation. The belief that the associate degree or diploma was a more desirable approach to becoming an RN was highly related to the students' beliefs that those educational routes were less costly. For some students, particularly those individuals with diplomas in nursing, the route to the baccalaureate is much longer and may be much more costly than it is for the student who chooses the generic degree. Certainly, issues of geographic access and financial resources to enter a bachelor's degree program may be barriers to initial preparation at the baccalaureate level. However, that RN students historically have not perceived the baccalaureate as initial preparation may have been due to the developmental context of nursing education at the time. For many of the RN students in this study, nonetheless, awareness that the investment will reap long-term rewards does appear to be present. These individuals seem to have realized that the nursing career requires further investment for greater potential rewards in the future.

Many students reported that the factors that affected their choice of a program were acceptance of transfer credits and convenient location. Access questions that relate to transfer of credit and opportunities for advanced standing are addressed in Chapter 4.

What is interesting is that students did not identify the availability of scholarships or grants as a key factor in choice of an RN/BSN program. RN students rely heavily on the tuition reimbursement programs provided by employers. Students in the study maintained close to full-time positions in nursing and worked an average of 32 hours a week. The important role played by employer tuition reimbursement programs was also noted in the previously cited cost study (Bednash, Redman, & Brinkman, 1989). In that study, the respondent RN students worked an average of 33 hours per week and used tuition reimbursement as a major source of support. Clearly, employers have made a commitment to a more educated work force and are an important support mechanism for the RN desiring to advance his or her education.

Cost can be an inhibiting factor in the selection of the bachelor's degree program as the initial preparation level, but it was not perceived as such by the respondents in this study who have made the choice to further their education by acquiring the bachelor's degree. However, it must be remembered that this study may not reflect the concerns of individuals who have not chosen to return for the bachelor's degree. For those individuals who have not reentered school to further their education, cost may indeed be inhibiting.

## REFERENCES

American Hospital Association. (1987). *Report of the Hospital Nursing Personnel Survey.* Chicago: Author.

American Nurses' Association. (1987). *The scope of nursing practice.* Kansas City, MO: Author.

Arlton, D. M. (1983). Academia: Learning the lay of the land. In D. L. Shane, (Ed.), *Returning to school,* Englewood Cliffs, NJ: Prentice-Hall.

Astin, A., Korn, W., & Green, K. C. (1987). Retaining and satisfying students. *Educational Record, 68*(1), 36–42.

Bednash, G., Redman, B., and Brinkman, P. (1989). *The economic investment in nursing education: Student, institutional, and clinical perspectives.* Washington, DC: Author.

Brainerd, N. S. (1983). From RN to BSN. *American Journal of Nursing,* *83*, 490.

Callin, M. (1983). Going back to school. *Journal of Continuing Education in Nursing, 14*(4), 21–27.

Cassells, J. M., Redman, B. K., & Jackson, S. S. (1986). Generic baccalaureate nursing student satisfaction regarding professional and personal development prior to graduation and one year post-graduation. *Journal of Professional Nursing, 2*, 114–127.

Griff, N. (1987). Meeting the career development needs of returning students. *Journal of College Student Personnel, 28*, 469–470.

Smith, D. L. (1986). *Costs of two levels of entry into nursing practice to nursing students, to health care consumers, and to institutions, for nursing education.* Bangor, ME: Maine State Nurses' Association.

Williams, J. R. (1984). Fears of the RN-BSN student. *Orthopedic Nursing, 3*, 49.

# 4
# Admission and Progression Through the Program

A description of policies, events, and experiences taken from the data on RN students' admission and progression through their programs provides important information about the content of RN/BSN education, instructional practices, time for completion, and student perceptions of growth and satisfaction with the program. Comparisons were made by type of program (incorporation into generic program, partial incorporation into generic program, RN separate track in generic program, or separate RN/BSN program).

This chapter focuses only minimally on adaptation to the program—a topic of considerable interest to RN students and to those involved with their education. The series of positive and negative emotional states believed to be experienced to some degree by all educationally mobile nurses enrolled in nursing programs has been described by one author as the returning-to-school-syndrome (Shane, 1983). It is thought to arise from role differences encountered in the nursing world the student knows best and the world of the educational program she/he enters. Its phases are described in Figure 4.1.

Although the usual progression is an irregular one, with relapses, detours, and expressways through certain stages, the experience generally begins with a brief honeymoon—a happy phase in which one's identity as a nurse is not being threatened and there is

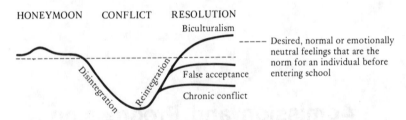

**Figure 4.1.** The returning-to-school syndrome: a model. From Shane, D. L. (1983). *Returning to school: A guide for nurses. Englewood Cliffs, NJ: Prentice-Hall.*

no expectation that one's performance as a nurse will change dramatically. The end of the honeymoon period comes with the first clinical nursing course, when one's self-image as a nurse is on the line. The RN student is then catapulted into Phase 2, which is characterized by conflict.

Phase 2 has a disintegration subphase followed by a reintegration subphase. In Phase III, the conflict is resolved in a variety of ways: through biculturalism, in which the nurse is a cosmopolitan citizen of several worlds in nursing; through false acceptance; through chronic conflict; and through oscillation from one resolution to another (Shane, 1983).

Both faculty and students must work at making a positive adjustment to this transition RN students experience. To facilitate a positive transition, many schools offer a bridge course as the first nursing course for RN students. Woolley (1984) describes the bridge course as providing orientation and overview of the curriculum students will be pursuing and how it relates to practice; as a demonstration of the conscious, continual application of theory as characteristic of the professional level of practice; and as important in aiding students to form their own peer group. Woolley discusses this model in greater detail in Chapter 7.

In fact, 61% of schools responding to this survey reported offering a bridge course, and most thought it was effective. Forty-three percent of students rated bridge courses between slightly and moderately effective as a tool for retention. Apparently, RN students do not perceive the bridge courses to be as useful as do the nurse educators in RN/BS programs. It would be interesting to study further the causes of these varying perspectives.

## ADMISSION AND ADVANCED PLACEMENT POLICIES

In the aggregate, admission decisions for RN students relied predominantly on prior grade point averages and less on standardized tests. Table 4.1 describes these requirements. It is also of interest to note that graduation from an NLN-accredited initial preparation program was required by nearly three fourths of the BSN programs surveyed. This requirement may be a result of the view held by many nurse educators that self-monitoring is inherent in a specialty

**TABLE 4.1. Deans' Report of Admission Requirements**

| Requirements/policies | Admission requirement | |
| --- | --- | --- |
| | No. | % |
| Current RN license in U.S | 396 | 86 |
| Current RN license in state where school is located | 327 | 71 |
| Graduate of NLN accredited nursing program (AD or diploma) | 340 | 73 |
| Prior cumulative GPA[a] | 341 | 74 |
| Nursing course GPA | 184 | 40 |
| Standardized NLN achievement tests | 96 | 21 |
| ACT exams | 84 | 18 |
| ACT-PEP exams | 74 | 16 |
| RN work experience required | 80 | 17 |
| Essay/writing test | 48 | 10 |
| SAT test | 38 | 8 |
| Language proficiency test if English not first language | 138 | 30 |

[a]GPA requirements using a 4.0 scale; 2.35, mean; 2.50, median.

accreditation review. Individuals who graduate from a program that has been accredited by the NLN have had an educational experience that has been shaped by standards of the profession. However, it must be noted that 29% of the respondents did not require this external validation of the original entry-level educational program.

Policies and procedures for recognizing and rewarding prior learning are known as advanced placement. One way to achieve advanced placement is to accept academic credits earned elsewhere. When credits are accepted for specific courses, the comparability of the courses must be established by the receiving institution; both the level and the content must be considered as well as how recently the student took the course. It is inappropriate to accept a lower-division course as comparable to an upper-division course (NLN, 1987).

A second way of establishing advanced placement is through awarding credit for prior learning through validation of a specific course or program objective (NLN, 1987). Awarding of credit without validating prior learning is inappropriate (COPA, 1979). The nursing program should conform to the parent institution's policies for admission, transferability of credits, design of a major, and degree requirements (AACN, 1986).

A previous study (Arlton & Miller, 1987) sampling only NLN-accredited baccalaureate nursing programs found that 95% of the programs provide an opportunity for RNs to obtain academic credit for prior learning in the nursing major, although the amount of credit that could be challenged varied greatly. The vast majority of programs were reported to assist students in preparing to take nursing challenge exams: 80% provide students with study guides and two thirds provide faculty counseling. A difference in practice was found by program type: 70% of generic programs admitting RNs use teacher-prepared exams for nursing theory, and only 39% of RN-only programs use this method of testing. The latter more frequently used the ACT-PEP tests (Arlton & Miller, 1987). These practices make sense because the generic programs must establish comparability of learning with already existing courses in the generic baccalaureate nursing curriculum.

Table 4-2 provides information about the variety of advanced-placement challenge exam methods reported by respondents in the present study.

**TABLE 4.2. Methods Used to Award Advanced Placement Credit (*n* = 461)**

| Method | No. of schools | % Schools |
|---|---|---|
| College Level Examination Program (CLEP) | 315 | 68.3 |
| American College Testing Proficiency Exam (ACT-PEP) | 275 | 59.7 |
| NLN exams | 192 | 41.6 |
| Teacher-made challenge exams | 176 | 38.2 |
| Clinical skills proficiency test | 143 | 31.0 |

Some states have regulated elements of curriculum and credit establishment policy. Ten percent of schools were in states that have regulations or statutes regarding credit for previous nursing education; schools reporting these regulations clustered in 15 states, and the number of credits so regulated averaged 35. Sixteen percent of schools reported state regulations or statutes about credit for previous non-nursing education. These schools were in 28 states, and the maximum number of non-nursing credits involved was, on the average, 61. Schools reported that 41 states have planning groups to discuss state policies regarding curriculum and credit requirements (see Table 4.3).

**TABLE 4.3. States with Regulations or Statutes Regarding Curriculum/Credit**

| Area | All states |
|---|---|
| State planning groups to discuss state policies regarding curriculum and credit requirements | 41 |
| Credit for previous nonnursing education | 28 |
| Curriculum requirements of RN baccalaureate education | 25 |
| Credit for previous nursing education | 15 |

## PATTERNS OF COURSEWORK

There are a number of questions of interest regarding coursework for the BSN. One question is what is required; a second is whether the content is integrated into a larger course or is presented as a separate course; third, whether the course can be challenged or transferred; and fourth, how graduates rate the degree of importance to clinical practice. Of course, there are many other valid reasons for taking coursework besides application to clinical practice.

The survey questions for the nursing subject matter were structured around the elements of *Essentials of College and University Education for Professional Nursing*, a report of the American Association of Colleges of Nursing (AACN, 1986). Besides describing general competencies that should be obtained from liberal education, the document makes explicit recommendations about the knowledge, skills, values, and professional behaviors to be included in programs preparing professional nurses. The "essentials" were derived by using a consensus-building model, and they describe the nursing profession's view of critical elements of education for professional practice. Thus, these elements are appropriate for use as a model to assess the RN student's learning during the bachelor's degree program. The entire *Essentials* document is reprinted in Appendix A.

Table 4.4 presents patterns of coursework reported for the liberal arts/sciences. Because questions asked in the 1984 survey of senior generic students (Cassells, Redman, & Jackson, 1986b) clustered subject matter in different ways, it was possible to make explicit comparisons of requirements reported by deans for RN/BSN programs in only a few areas (see Table 4.5). Instruction was least frequently required in economics and foreign languages and to a lesser extent in political science, computer technology, anthropology, and management. Differences may be ascribed to different times for collection of the data, different sources (senior students, deans), or different respondents in particular RN-only programs.

Although most of this content was taught in separate courses, pharmacology, pathophysiology, and, to lesser extent, nutrition were most commonly integrated. University policy allows transfer and, to some degree, challenge of many of these subjects. Actual reported experience of students shows low levels of activity in challenging these subjects and high levels of transfer, especially in psychology, microbiology, sociology, anatomy, physiology, and English composition. Nutrition (14%) and pharmacology (15%) were the most frequently challenged. At 6 months postgraduation, RN student respondents saw much of the science/mathematical curriculum as highly important in clinical nursing, especially anatomy and physiology, pharmacology, pathophysiology, and nutrition. In the social sciences, psychology, sociology, and growth and development were perceived as very important, as were ethics, speech, and English composition in the humanities/liberal arts. Further, management was perceived as very important.

Table 4.6 presents similar information on nursing subject matter. The findings presented again provide information about whether the content was required, integrated or taught in a separate course, challengeable, or transferrable. In addition, estimates by deans and students of the emphasis on these elements during the program, and new graduates' estimates of skill level and of application of the skill/knowledge in clinical practice 6 months postgraduation, are reported.

The norm was for most schools to require students to complete or show evidence of the knowledge/skills in order to graduate. Exceptions to this included international health and computer-information processing principles/skills and what might be considered specialized areas of practice, such as occupational health, critical care, perioperative care, and emergency care. The baccalaureate is still considered to prepare a generalist in nursing. It is interesting to note that although computer education has been stressed as necessary in nursing education, only half of the graduates report application of this knowledge/skill in the clinical setting.

Nursing research, physical assessment, and community health were frequently reported as being taught in separate courses; most of the rest of the content is reported as being integrated into more broadly based courses. With the exception of physical assessment, most of these content elements showed low levels of challengeability/transferability, probably in part because they do not represent courselike bundles of knowledge and skills. Medical-surgical (adult health), pediatrics, ob-gyn/women's health, and

**TABLE 4.4. Patterns of Coursework in the Liberal Arts and Rated Importance to Clinical Practice**

| Content | How content can be acquired Deans (n = 461) | | | | | % RN students reporting challenge/transfer (n = 742) | | | Mean rating 6 mo. postgraduation of importance in clinical nursing (n = 427)[a] |
|---|---|---|---|---|---|---|---|---|---|
| | % R | % I | % S | % C | % T | % C | % T | % DNH | |
| Scientific/mathematical | | | | | | | | | |
| Mathematics | 53.1 | 6.7 | 54.0 | 38.2 | 57.0 | 5.5 | 37.6 | 27.9 | 2.77 |
| Statistics | 65.5 | 3.9 | 69.4 | 23.9 | 70.3 | .9 | 17.9 | 21.0 | 2.45 |
| Biology | 41.9 | 4.1 | 49.5 | 27.8 | 51.8 | 3.8 | 51.3 | 24.0 | 3.21 |
| Microbiology | 86.1 | 2.8 | 78.7 | 49.5 | 83.9 | 5.4 | 70.6 | 3.0 | 3.25 |
| Anatomy & physiology | 89.6 | 3.3 | 79.6 | 53.1 | 84.6 | 8.8 | 67.1 | 2.2 | 3.76 |
| Chemistry | 87.4 | 2.2 | 80.9 | 47.5 | 85.7 | 2.3 | 55.0 | 3.4 | 2.68 |
| Nutrition | 64.0 | 19.3 | 57.3 | 44.9 | 64.6 | 13.7 | 46.1 | 16.8 | 3.49 |
| Pharmacology | 46.2 | 33.6 | 37.7 | 30.8 | 43.6 | 14.7 | 33.2 | 30.6 | 3.73 |
| Pathophysiology | 56.4 | 27.3 | 45.3 | 28.0 | 44.5 | 8.1 | 19.9 | 25.2 | 3.74 |
| Social sciences | | | | | | | | | |
| Psychology | 87.2 | 2.2 | 79.0 | 51.6 | 85.9 | 3.6 | 72.2 | 1.9 | 3.57 |
| Sociology | 84.6 | 2.2 | 78.3 | 49.7 | 84.6 | 2.7 | 71.3 | 3.5 | 3.22 |
| Growth & development | 77.7 | 12.1 | 68.3 | 44.7 | 76.4 | 10.5 | 51.5 | 8.1 | 3.36 |

| | | | | | | | | | |
|---|---|---|---|---|---|---|---|---|---|
| Anthropology | 24.5 | 4.8 | 38.6 | 12.1 | 42.7 | .1 | 17.9 | 58.8 | 2.36 |
| Economics | 10.8 | 6.1 | 33.2 | 10.4 | 34.5 | .3 | 11.3 | 78.8 | 2.60 |
| Political Science | 23.2 | 4.1 | 42.1 | 14.8 | 43.6 | .5 | 23.7 | 60.4 | 2.10 |
| Humanities/liberal arts | | | | | | | | | |
| Philosophy, logic | 45.1 | 3.7 | 53.4 | 15.4 | 57.0 | .7 | 24.5 | 36.4 | 2.62 |
| Religion | 33.6 | 3.9 | 45.1 | 11.3 | 46.0 | .5 | 14.8 | 54.9 | 2.65 |
| Ethics | 34.5 | 16.5 | 38.6 | 11.7 | 44.7 | 1.1 | 13.6 | 44.7 | 3.51 |
| English composition | 89.8 | 1.1 | 80.7 | 11.3 | 86.1 | 4.7 | 65.1 | 2.6 | 3.13 |
| Literature/classics | 58.4 | 1.5 | 61.8 | 29.5 | 65.7 | 4.2 | 41.2 | 19.0 | 2.22 |
| Speech | 37.1 | 3.0 | 48.2 | 16.7 | 50.8 | 1.2 | 34.8 | 39.2 | 3.12 |
| Foreign language | 11.3 | .7 | 32.3 | 13.2 | 33.2 | 1.3 | 17.9 | 69.4 | 2.29 |
| History/geography | 51.4 | .9 | 57.9 | 27.1 | 60.3 | 2.4 | 40.4 | 26.1 | 1.87 |
| Other studies | | | | | | | | | |
| Management | 25.8 | 12.6 | 31.5 | 9.3 | 28.4 | 2.2 | 5.7 | 37.5 | 3.45 |
| Computer technology | 23.6 | 6.9 | 35.6 | 9.5 | 36.7 | .4 | 5.3 | 69.7 | 3.10 |
| Research | 57.3 | 12.6 | 51.0 | 11.9 | 37.5 | 1.5 | 3.0 | 14.6 | 2.88 |

R, required; I, integrated; S, separate course; C, challengeable; T, transferable; DNH, did not have.
[a] 1, not important; 2, minimally important; 3, moderately important; 4, very important.

**TABLE 4.5.  Non-nursing Content/Course Requirements for BSN Degree**

| Requirements | 1984 generic students (% required) | 1987 deans reported requirements for RN students (% required) |
|---|---|---|
| Anthropology | 62 | 25 |
| Computer technology | 26 | 59 |
| Economics | 32 | 11 |
| Psychology | 95 | 87 |
| Sociology | 85 | 89 |
| Speech | 73 | 37 |

psychiatric/mental health nursing were most frequently reported as being challengeable or transferrable, perhaps in part because they do represent courselike bundles of knowledge and skills.

The data show that different estimate scales exist for program emphasis by deans and students. On most content items, there was agreement on the estimates of deans and students, and most showed a high degree of emphasis. This finding is congruent with the finding of the *Essentials* project, that is, a high degree of consensus on nearly all of the skills, knowledge, and values identified as essential (AACN, 1986). Content reported by deans to be receiving between slightly low and slightly high emphasis or reported by students as moderate emphasis included international health, occupational health issues/needs, and computer-information processing principles/skills (see Table 4.6). Students also reported that change theory principles received moderate emphasis.

Students reported being between moderately and very skilled in most content areas. On the average, students rated themselves as minimally skilled in computer information processing principles/skills and slightly more skilled in international health principles/issues. Low ratings of computer skills were also found for new generic graduates surveyed in 1985 (Cassells, Redman, & Jackson,

1986a). Ratings by new RN/BSN graduates of their application of content in clinical settings contained one surprise: the relatively low level of use of theories/models of nursing practice. That finding is of concern because many baccalaureate programs emphasize that element as important to professional nursing practice. The content area most frequently applied by new RN/BSN graduates 6 months after completion of the program was the nursing process.

The data in Table 4.7 provide gross comparisons of the reported application by new generic graduates and new RN/BSN graduates of three key nursing concepts (Cassells et al., 1986a).

Students provided perceptions of their knowledge/skill levels in all areas represented in Table 4.6 on entering and on exiting from the BSN program. In all areas, their perceptions of their growth were highly significant ($p < .001$ using a matched $t$ test); the $t$ values ranged from $-57.56$ to $-18.31$. Using mean differences, the greatest perceived changes in skill levels occurred in community health, gerontology, and infectious/communicable disease care. Interestingly, when mean differences were placed in rank order, the greatest perceived changes in knowledge/skill occurred in the areas of nursing research, theories/models of nursing practice, nursing diagnosis, change theory principles, trends and issues in nursing, and the nursing process. Therefore, although RN/BSN graduates reported that the greatest change in knowledge/skill occurs in theories/models of nursing practice, little applicability of this content was perceived by the graduates. This may be reflective of the inflexibility in the practice environment and its poor differentiation of the professional nursing role. However, it may also be a result of poor articulation, by nursing educators, of the applicability of nursing theories/models to nursing practice.

Also of interest was the kind of clinical courses/experiences required of RN students. Table 4.8 presents information about the degree to which a clinical experience in a variety of settings is required, the degree to which these courses/experiences can be challenged or transferred, and the kind of student supervision used. The data show a large percentage of schools requiring experience in community health. Some settings were used relatively little (HMOs, boardinghouses, hospices) or may not be available. Oppor-

TABLE 4.6. Patterns of Coursework/Content in Nursing and Graduate-Rated Skill/Application to Clinical Practice

| | Dean (n=461) Content/course requirements | | | | | Emphasis | | Graduating students estimate of skill level n=742 (mean)c | % Graduating students reporting application in clinical setting 6 mo. post-graduation n=427 |
| | % R | % I | % S | % C | % T | Dean n=461 (mean)a | Student n=742 (mean)b | | |
|---|---|---|---|---|---|---|---|---|---|
| GENERAL | | | | | | | | | |
| Nursing process | 90.5 | 78.7 | 10.6 | 27.3 | 23.0 | 5.80 | 3.89 | 3.59 | 81.3 |
| Nursing diagnosis | 89.4 | 82.4 | 3.7 | 24.9 | 19.1 | 5.62 | 3.82 | 3.54 | 70.5 |
| Theories/models of nursing practice | 86.6 | 70.7 | 14.3 | 14.5 | 16.3 | 4.81 | 3.69 | 3.05 | 31.4 |
| Historical aspects of nursing | 80.7 | 69.6 | 11.3 | 18.7 | 19.7 | 4.00 | 3.03 | 2.79 | 13.3 |
| Nursing research | 90.7 | 23.4 | 68.5 | 15.4 | 32.8 | 5.46 | 3.74 | 3.08 | 44.5 |
| Standards of nursing practice | 86.3 | 83.5 | 2.6 | 14.8 | 14.1 | 5.08 | 3.60 | 3.30 | 82.7 |
| Ethics of nursing practice | 87.0 | 76.4 | 13.0 | 13.9 | 16.3 | 5.36 | 3.53 | 3.37 | 85.2 |
| Trends and Issues in nursing | 89.8 | 46.2 | 44.0 | 16.3 | 24.1 | 5.17 | 3.62 | 3.33 | 71.9 |
| Physical assessment skills | 89.4 | 33.0 | 59.0 | 33.0 | 35.8 | 5.49 | 3.61 | 3.46 | 81.3 |
| SUPPORTIVE/ENVIRONMENTAL KNOWLEDGE | | | | | | | | | |
| Wellness and health promotion | 86.1 | 79.2 | 10.0 | 19.1 | 14.8 | 5.58 | 3.77 | 3.45 | 81.3 |

| | | | | | | | | |
|---|---|---|---|---|---|---|---|---|
| Human spirituality principles/needs | 69.0 | 75.3 | 3.5 | 14.3 | 11.3 | 4.38 | 3.14 | 3.07 | 78.9 |
| Cross cultural issues/principles | 80.9 | 81.8 | 5.6 | 15.4 | 12.8 | 4.71 | 3.31 | 2.96 | 67.4 |
| International health principles/issues | 45.8 | 57.0 | 3.9 | 9.3 | 8.7 | 3.45 | 2.61 | 2.25 | 25.3 |
| Family & group dynamic principles | 85.5 | 73.3 | 15.8 | 18.2 | 14.8 | 5.36 | 3.65 | 3.28 | 78.2 |
| Health care delivery principles | 85.2 | 77.4 | 11.9 | 13.2 | 12.8 | 5.13 | 3.55 | 3.18 | 77.3 |
| Legal/legislative principles/issues | 85.2 | 78.1 | 12.4 | 13.2 | 13.0 | 5.02 | 3.42 | 3.06 | 67.7 |
| Political principles/issues | 81.3 | 76.1 | 10.8 | 10.4 | 11.5 | 4.69 | 3.15 | 2.79 | 45.9 |
| Ethical principles/issues | 84.8 | 76.4 | 14.3 | 13.2 | 13.4 | 5.26 | 3.50 | 3.27 | 82.7 |
| Economic/cost containment: principles/issues | 73.1 | 75.5 | 5.4 | 9.8 | 10.2 | 4.36 | 3.08 | 2.96 | 75.9 |
| Occupational health issues/needs | 65.9 | 70.9 | 3.5 | 8.7 | 8.2 | 3.83 | 2.87 | 2.58 | 48.7 |
| INTEGRATIVE/KNOWLEDGE SKILLS | | | | | | | | | |
| Physiological alterations | 85.5 | 70.9 | 16.7 | 26.0 | 18.2 | 5.39 | 3.50 | 3.37 | 87.1 |
| Psychological alterations | 85.2 | 75.5 | 11.7 | 24.3 | 15.8 | 5.37 | 3.54 | 3.31 | 87.4 |
| Social alterations | 83.1 | 78.1 | 5.9 | 20.6 | 13.7 | 5.15 | 3.48 | 3.23 | 83.6 |
| ADAPTIVE KNOWLEDGE/SKILLS | | | | | | | | | |
| Organizational principles/skills | 84.2 | 61.2 | 29.3 | 11.7 | 14.3 | 5.14 | 3.35 | 3.34 | 85.0 |
| Management principles/skills | 86.3 | 50.8 | 39.3 | 12.6 | 15.6 | 5.27 | 3.55 | 3.28 | 75.6 |

**TABLE 4.6.** (continued)

| | Dean (n = 461) Content/course requirements | | | | | Emphasis | | Graduating students estimate of skill level n = 742 (mean)[c] | % Graduating students reporting application in clinical setting 6 mo. post-graduation n = 427 |
| | % R | % I | % S | % C | % T | Dean n = 461 (mean)[a] | Student n = 742 (mean)[b] | | |
| --- | --- | --- | --- | --- | --- | --- | --- | --- | --- |
| Leadership principles/skills | 86.6 | 53.6 | 36.9 | 11.9 | 14.3 | 5.50 | 3.70 | 3.41 | 83.6 |
| Assertiveness principles/skills | 73.8 | 74.2 | 8.5 | 9.5 | 10.2 | 4.81 | 3.43 | 3.31 | 88.1 |
| Setting priorities principles/skills | 83.3 | 79.8 | 6.5 | 10.8 | 10.8 | 5.25 | 3.39 | 3.47 | 89.0 |
| Teaching/learning principles/skills | 85.7 | 76.6 | 11.9 | 13.4 | 13.0 | 5.44 | 3.68 | 3.45 | 86.7 |
| Crisis intervention/stress management principles/skills | 82.9 | 77.9 | 7.8 | 13.0 | 11.1 | 5.01 | 3.33 | 3.18 | 82.2 |
| Change theory principles | 83.5 | 74.6 | 10.8 | 10.0 | 10.4 | 5.04 | 2.15 | 2.97 | 66.0 |
| Computer-information processing principles/skills | 39.0 | 34.7 | 20.2 | 6.5 | 13.0 | 3.62 | 2.17 | 2.06 | 46.4 |

## COMMUNICATION

| | | | | | | | | | Mean** |
|---|---|---|---|---|---|---|---|---|---|
| Supervision of nursing care | 76.1 | 68.8 | 10.0 | 9.5 | 8.7 | 4.90 | 3.10 | 3.24 | 78.7 |
| Documentation of concise data using standard terminology | 79.4 | 78.3 | 2.0 | 13.7 | 10.2 | 5.18 | 3.26 | 3.39 | 87.6 |
| Collaboration with client/health care providers to establish mutual client objectives/goals | 84.6 | 82.2 | 2.6 | 11.9 | 9.3 | 5.43 | 3.47 | 3.27 | 80.3 |
| Use of interdisciplinary resources/relationship(s) | 82.4 | 81.8 | 1.5 | 11.1 | 9.3 | 5.10 | 3.46 | 3.31 | 83.6 |
| Promotion of group dynamics | 83.9 | 78.1 | 7.4 | 11.3 | 9.5 | 5.25 | 3.49 | 3.14 | 71.0 |

## SPECIFIC CLINICAL AREAS

| | | | | | | | | | Mean** |
|---|---|---|---|---|---|---|---|---|---|
| Medical-surgical | 81.0 | 37.0 | 41.0 | 58.0 | 27.0 | 5.30 | 3.30 | 3.46 | 3.66[d] |
| Pediatric care | 78.0 | 40.0 | 35.0 | 60.0 | 26.0 | 5.10 | 2.90 | 2.76 | 3.18[d] |
| Obstetric/gynecologic care | 76.0 | 40.0 | 31.0 | 57.0 | 25.0 | 5.00 | 2.80 | 2.83 | 3.18[d] |
| Psychiatric care | 80.0 | 36.0 | 38.0 | 54.0 | 24.0 | 5.20 | 3.10 | 2.90 | 3.33[d] |
| Community health | 89.0 | 25.0 | 62.0 | 17.0 | 20.0 | 5.80 | 3.90 | 3.33 | 3.48[d] |
| Gerontology | 68.0 | 70.0 | 11.0 | 24.0 | 17.0 | 4.80 | 3.00 | 2.99 | 3.67[d] |
| Long-term care | 63.0 | 67.0 | 6.0 | 22.0 | 13.0 | 4.50 | 2.80 | 2.82 | 3.19[d] |
| Critical care | 52.0 | 49.0 | 14.0 | 23.0 | 13.0 | 4.40 | 2.70 | 2.85 | 3.28[d] |
| Cardiovascular | 64.0 | 69.0 | 4.0 | 30.0 | 15.0 | 4.70 | 2.90 | 3.04 | 3.40[d] |
| Infectious/communicable care | 63.0 | 70.0 | 3.0 | 22.0 | 15.0 | 4.40 | 2.90 | 2.88 | 3.34[d] |
| Rehabilitation | 63.0 | 67.0 | 7.0 | 22.0 | 14.0 | 4.50 | 2.70 | 2.59 | 3.11[d] |

**TABLE 4.6.** (continued)

| | Dean (n=461) Content/course requirements | | | | | | Emphasis | | Graduating students estimate of skill level n=742 (mean)[c] | % Graduating students reporting application in clinical setting 6 mo. post-graduation n=427 |
| | | | | | | | Dean n=461 (mean)[a] | Student n=742 (mean)[b] | | |
| | % R | % I | % S | % C | % T | | | | | |
| Perioperative care | 50.0 | 59.0 | 4.0 | 29.0 | 16.0 | | 4.20 | 2.30 | 2.71 | 2.96[d] |
| Emergency care | 44.0 | 58.0 | 4.0 | 21.0 | 13.0 | | 3.80 | 2.40 | 2.74 | 3.21[d] |

R, required; I, integrated; S, separated; C, challengeable; T, transferrable.

[a]Emphasis on deans' scale was 1 to 6: 1, very low; 2, moderately low; 3, slightly low; 4, slightly high; 5, moderately high; 6, very high.

[b]Emphasis on students' scale was 1 to 4: 1, none; 2, low; 3, moderate; 4, high.

[c]1, not skilled; 2, minimally skilled; 3, moderately skilled; 4, very skilled.

[d]RN students were asked to rate the degree of importance in applying nursing content to clinical practice upon completion of their BSN coursework, not 6 months after graduation as in the other areas: 1, not important; 2, minimally important; 3, moderately important; 4, very important.

TABLE 4.7. **Comparisons of Three Key Nursing Concepts**

|  | % Generic graduates reporting application at 12 months postgraduation ($n$ = 432) | % RN/BSN graduates reporting application at 6 months postgraduation ($n$ = 426) |
|---|---|---|
| Nursing process | 86 | 81 |
| Nursing theories/models | 51 | 31 |
| Nursing diagnosis | 87 | 71 |

tunities for challenge seemed to be most available in the content associated with traditional core areas of acute-care settings.

Although estimates of the type of supervision provided, by deans and by students, differed somewhat in magnitude, some patterns are discernible. Again, direct faculty supervision was most likely to occur in community health, traditional acute-care settings, and home-care settings. There was a relatively strong use of preceptors, which deans feel to be quite effective, and, to a lesser extent, independently arranged clinical experience.

Deans reported a mean clinical supervision ratio of 1 faculty member to 9.25 RN students. Sixty-three percent of them also reported use of contractual agreements between faculty and RN students, and 80% reported RN student use of the learning resource center.

For many of these settings, a high percentage of students reported not having clinical experience (see Tables 4.4, 4.6, and 4.8). Because students responded to the surveys in February or March and expected to graduate by June, it is unlikely that they would have added to their clinical experiences by the time of graduation. Perhaps students are defining clinical experience narrowly, or perhaps educators were using the student's work environment as a clinical laboratory experience. Still, these data suggest the need for further study of the character of clinical experience for RN students.

Students perceived that they had grown the most in knowledge

**TABLE 4.8. Patterns of Clinical Experience Setting Use and Supervision**

| Clinical course/experience | Deans (n = 461) | | | Type of supervision reported by deans (n = 461) | | | Type of supervision reported by students (n = 742) | | | % not having clinical experience (n = 472) |
|---|---|---|---|---|---|---|---|---|---|---|
| | % R | % C | % T | % D | % P | % I | % D | % P | % I | |
| Acute-care setting | | | | | | | | | | |
| Medical-surgical | 64.2 | 39.5 | 18.2 | 49.0 | 18.2 | 5.0 | 30.6 | 6.2 | 9.4 | 51.1 |
| Psychiatric care | 57.5 | 35.1 | 16.3 | 43.0 | 17.4 | 4.3 | 23.0 | 5.7 | 8.4 | 60.9 |
| Pediatric care | 55.3 | 39.3 | 18.2 | 40.3 | 16.1 | 3.7 | 20.2 | 3.4 | 6.2 | 68.1 |
| Obstetric/gynecologic care | 54.2 | 39.0 | 18.7 | 38.8 | 15.4 | 3.9 | 18.2 | 5.4 | 5.5 | 69.0 |
| Cardiovascular | 42.5 | 22.6 | 13.4 | 36.2 | 16.5 | 4.3 | 18.6 | 9.7 | 6.9 | 63.6 |
| Rehabilitation | 38.6 | 15.8 | 11.5 | 29.1 | 16.3 | 5.2 | 16.2 | 4.7 | 5.9 | 70.9 |
| Intensive care | 31.5 | 15.6 | 9.8 | 29.9 | 18.2 | 3.7 | 15.0 | 10.5 | 4.7 | 68.7 |
| Infectious/communicable care | 30.6 | 13.7 | 11.3 | 24.5 | 14.8 | 5.4 | 16.4 | 5.3 | 7.0 | 69.1 |
| Emergency care | 22.8 | 11.5 | 8.7 | 19.5 | 17.8 | 4.1 | 84.0 | 7.0 | 4.7 | 78.2 |

Ambulatory-care setting

| | | | | | | | | | |
|---|---|---|---|---|---|---|---|---|---|
| Wellness/screening clinic | 54.7 | 10.4 | 9.3 | 38.2 | 23.9 | 9.1 | 25.6 | 16.7 | 12.4 | 44.1 |
| General clinic | 32.3 | 7.6 | 7.4 | 22.1 | 19.1 | 4.8 | 14.8 | 11.1 | 6.3 | 62.0 |
| Psychiatric outpatient | 28.9 | 9.8 | 6.5 | 22.8 | 17.4 | 6.1 | 8.0 | 4.4 | 4.2 | 80.3 |
| Acute-care clinic | 24.3 | 8.9 | 7.6 | 17.8 | 17.4 | 6.1 | 9.6 | 5.3 | 4.2 | 77.9 |
| Outpatient surgery care clinic | 13.9 | 6.3 | 6.1 | 12.8 | 18.0 | 5.0 | 5.0 | 3.8 | 3.8 | 85.2 |
| Other nonhospital setting | | | | | | | | | | |
| Community health | 83.7 | 9.8 | 10.8 | 64.4 | 28.0 | 7.6 | 47.0 | 28.6 | 17.3 | 9.2 |
| Home care agencies | 52.7 | 6.9 | 7.4 | 36.7 | 26.5 | 7.4 | 22.1 | 25.1 | 15.2 | 37.6 |
| Long-term care/ nursing home | 31.5 | 10.4 | 7.6 | 28.6 | 13.4 | 6.1 | 11.7 | 2.6 | 6.7 | 76.7 |
| School nurse | 25.4 | 4.3 | 5.2 | 15.4 | 24.9 | 7.8 | 8.2 | 16.3 | 10.5 | 62.8 |
| Rehabilitation center | 18.2 | 5.2 | 4.3 | 17.6 | 15.6 | 5.2 | 10.1 | 3.6 | 5.4 | 78.2 |
| Volunteer agencies | 15.2 | 3.7 | 3.9 | 8.0 | 17.1 | 8.9 | 5.3 | 5.0 | 13.6 | 73.5 |
| Hospice | 10.2 | 3.0 | 3.9 | 8.5 | 18.7 | 6.1 | 5.4 | 6.6 | 7.1 | 77.9 |
| HMO | 4.8 | 2.4 | 3.7 | 5.0 | 12.6 | 5.4 | 1.3 | 2.2 | 2.2 | 90.2 |
| Geriatric setting | | | | | | | | | | |
| Community health agency | 64.6 | 7.6 | 8.7 | 50.1 | 20.4 | 9.3 | 33.7 | 20.5 | 14.4 | 30.3 |
| Home care agency | 47.9 | 6.9 | 7.2 | 33.8 | 21.5 | 8.0 | 17.7 | 18.9 | 12.7 | 49.3 |
| Acute-care facility | 40.1 | 12.1 | 9.3 | 35.8 | 13.7 | 3.5 | 22.9 | 6.2 | 8.0 | 60.8 |
| Long-term care | 29.5 | 6.5 | 5.6 | 26.2 | 14.8 | 6.1 | 10.2 | 3.1 | 5.0 | 77.2 |
| Nursing homes | 28.9 | 10.2 | 7.8 | 28.6 | 12.6 | 4.8 | 10.6 | 2.4 | 5.7 | 78.7 |

**TABLE 4.8.** (continued)

| Clinical course/experience | Deans (n = 461) | | | Type of supervision reported by deans (n = 461) | | | Type of supervision reported by students (n = 742) | | | % not having clinical experience (n = 472) |
|---|---|---|---|---|---|---|---|---|---|---|
| | % R | % C | % T | % D | % P | % I | % D | % P | % I | |
| Senior citizens center | 21.7 | 5.4 | 5.0 | 16.5 | 13.4 | 10.6 | 11.6 | 5.4 | 12.0 | 67.9 |
| Geriatric day-care center | 15.2 | 4.1 | 4.1 | 11.3 | 14.1 | 8.5 | 7.5 | 4.0 | 6.3 | 79.0 |
| Retirement facility | 14.8 | 4.1 | 4.1 | 12.4 | 12.8 | 7.4 | 5.8 | 2.2 | 5.9 | 83.3 |
| Boardinghouse (SRO) | 3.0 | 2.0 | 3.0 | 4.8 | 8.9 | 5.6 | 1.2 | .8 | 2.6 | 92.0 |

R, required; C, challenged; T, transferred; D, direct faculty; P, preceptor; I, independent.

and skill in the community health area, including geriatric community health. Students' ratings of their levels of skill and knowledge at the beginning of their programs and at the end were significantly different ($p < .001$) in all settings. It is particularly significant that students reported an enhanced level of skills and knowledge regarding the geriatric patient. This patient group is growing and constitutes a major focus for health care professionals.

Deans reported a mean of 7.4 hours of academic advisement per student per year, and RN students reported a mean of 8.2 hours per year. In 40% of the schools, advisement was conducted by a faculty member designated as the RN advisor, 36% divided RN students among faculty, and 6% reported hiring an adviser solely to advise RN students.

## TRANSITION THROUGH THE PROGRAM

As has been noted earlier, a high percentage of RN students went to school part-time and continued to work. Data in the senior student sample showed that during the year 1985–86, 50% attended school part-time, 34% attended full-time, and an additional 16% combined of part-time and full-time attendance. These same students showed slightly different patterns for 1986–87, with 45% attending school full-time.

On the average, deans reported that it takes a student 2 years (with a standard deviation of 0.6 year) to complete the program if attending full-time and 3.7 years (with a standard deviation of 1.1 years) if attending part-time. Sixty percent of deans reported that their institutions have no time limit within which RN students must complete the program. Thirteen percent reported an average maximum time limit of 5 years, and an additional 28% reported that a maximum time limit exists but waiver is permitted. These findings are corroborated by a recent cost study completed by the American Association of Colleges of Nursing (Bednash, Redman, & Brinkman, 1989). This study found that RN students required, on the average, 3.6 years to complete the bachelor's degree while attending part-time. Further, the RN students in the cost study were most likely to be working, as noted earlier, and maintaining a nursing position.

To get a sense of program completion rate, deans were asked what percentage of the RN students who had enrolled for the first time in 1978–79 had graduated by August 1986. The mean of their responses was 86% with a standard deviation of 19%, and the median was 94%. Factors that deans felt strongly influenced noncompletion rates included personal reasons, inadequate financial support, and conflict with employment schedules. They rated the following factors as slightly important to noncompletion rates: academic program too difficult, resistance to socialization to the student role, frustration with curriculum requirements, and unrealistic expectations. Incompatibility with the program's philosophy, being counseled by the school to withdraw, and lack of peer support were thought to be very unimportant reasons for noncompletion. Deans' perceptions of the importance of reasons for noncompletion did not differ by program type except for student frustration with curriculum requirements, which was rated as more common in programs in which RNs were integrated with generic students than in RN completion programs [$F$ (3, 353) = 5.56, $p < .001$]. Therefore, it is interesting to note that although deans may perceive peer support to be relatively unimportant in relation to a student's ability to complete a program, students' frustrations with curriculum requirements are more enhanced in a program that requires integration with generic students. The RN/BSN student may be responding with frustration to the need to complete requirements similar to those for generic students and also may be frustrated simply because fewer peers are available to provide support.

Both deans and students agreed that the following strategies were very to moderately effective in helping RN students complete their program: providing schedule flexibility to accommodate working students, providing specific academic advisors for RN students, modifying clinical requirements according to students' work experience, offering courses off-campus, offering RN-only courses, tailoring course requirements, and preparing faculty to meet specific learning needs of RN students. Students rated peer support as the most important retention strategy. Again, it is important to note that students do rate peer support as extremely important to retention, in contrast with the perceptions held by deans. Perhaps greater attention to peer groups and the use of support activities by peers will increase retention, and potentially recruitment, of additional RNs in the baccalaureate program.

## STUDENT PERCEPTIONS OF GROWTH AND CAREER PLANS

Because the BSN was a second stage of professional development through education for these students, it is important to understand how they felt about their growth at a time when they were nearing completion of the program. Data about student perceptions of their own growth are presented in Table 4.9. In general, they showed average scores tending toward moderate improvement, particularly strong in research capabilities, preparation for graduate or professional school, confidence in academic abilities, and general academic knowledge. Students' estimates of their growth in nursing knowledge and in clinical judgment and decision making were slightly lower. For all areas of growth there was considerable variability among students, but in a number of areas there was a consistent tendency for those indicating moderate and, especially, great improvement in their personal and professional growth to be in programs that separated RN students from generic students.

Student satisfaction with structural components and practices of their programs is also important. Data presented in Table 4.10 show that requirements for courses were rated better than moderately adequate, as were the number of non-nursing courses transferred. The least satisfaction was with number of clinical hours transferred and challenged. Again, there was considerable variability in students' ratings. Students liked elective clinical experiences, independent learning contracts, patient teaching projects, and the preceptor system for instruction in clinical agencies and thought that they were effective.

Students were asked to project in what type of setting and in what area of nursing they would be working 10 years hence. It is noteworthy that although more than half of the students had been most recently employed in hospitals and one third of them planned to work in hospitals after completing the BSN, only one quarter wanted to be working in hospitals in 10 years. Nine percent wanted

**TABLE 4.9. RN Students' Perceptions of Professional and Personal Growth Since Entering the BSN Program (n = 742)**

| Area | No. | Mean[a] | SD |
|---|---|---|---|
| Research capabilities | 729 | 3.15 | .82 |
| Confidence in academic abilities | 728 | 3.14 | .91 |
| Preparation for graduate/professional school | 733 | 3.14 | .81 |
| General academic knowledge | 728 | 3.12 | .76 |
| Motivation to continue education after graduation | 725 | 3.00 | 1.00 |
| Ability to identify strength and weaknesses | 727 | 2.97 | .93 |
| Cultural awareness and appreciation | 732 | 2.92 | .91 |
| Leadership abilities | 732 | 2.91 | .89 |
| General knowledge about living, life, self | 730 | 2.91 | .89 |
| Analytical and problem-solving skills | 730 | 2.90 | .86 |
| Nursing knowledge in general | 724 | 2.90 | .78 |
| Attitudes, values, and personal qualities (curiosity, ethical integrity, intellectual drive, humaneness, emotional stability) | 733 | 2.84 | .98 |
| Ability to speak and write clearly | 730 | 2.77 | .96 |
| Ability to work independently | 730 | 2.74 | 1.08 |
| Clinical judgment and decision making | 728 | 2.69 | .97 |
| Job search skills | 729 | 2.43 | 1.01 |

[a]1, no change; 2, minimal improvement; 3, moderate improvement; 4, great improvement.

to be working in schools of nursing; 10%, in independent practice; 8%, in community health agencies; 4%, in home health; 2%, in nursing homes/gerontology settings; and 2%, in military nursing. A number were undecided. These responses are startling.

The fact that few RN students wanted to remain in the acute care setting post-BSN raises questions about the perceived attractiveness of this work environment. Generic students also reported that only 39% expected to be working in hospitals in 10 years

**TABLE 4.10. RN Students' Perceptions about the Adequacy of BSN Program Components (*n* = 742)**

| Component | No. | Mean[a] | SD |
|---|---|---|---|
| Number of nursing course hours required | 716 | 5.34 | 1.03 |
| Number of non-nursing hours required | 710 | 5.30 | 1.01 |
| Number of clinical hours required | 700 | 5.11 | 1.37 |
| Courses taken with RNs only | 614 | 5.10 | 1.39 |
| Number of non-nursing course hours transferred | 653 | 5.06 | 1.34 |
| Sites of clinical experience | 698 | 4.65 | 1.41 |
| Number of non-nursing course hours challenged | 404 | 4.52 | 1.57 |
| Faculty advisement throughout the baccalaureate program | 713 | 4.48 | 1.68 |
| Bridge or transition courses required | 442 | 4.44 | 1.43 |
| Relevance of clinical practice coursework | 704 | 4.42 | 1.52 |
| Number of nursing course hours challenged | 508 | 4.39 | 1.69 |
| Courses taken with generic students | 433 | 4.39 | 1.59 |
| Number of nursing course hours transferred | 554 | 3.94 | 2.04 |
| Number of clinical hours challenged | 387 | 3.78 | 1.93 |
| Number of clinical hours transferred | 476 | 3.58 | 2.13 |

1, very inaquate; 2, moderately inadequate; 3, slightly inadequate; 4, slightly adequate; 5, moderately adequate; 6, very adequate.

(Cassells et al., 1986b). In addition, as noted earlier, many RNs return to acquire the BS degree as a stepping-stone to the master's degree or other advanced education. The fact that certain percentages of these returning RNs desire a postbaccalaureate career as nurse educators or independent practitioners identifies their goals for the advanced degree(s). Currently, much of the publicity surrounding the nursing shortage has focused on RN vacancy rates in the acute-care setting. The strong indication by RNs returning for the bachelor's degree, as well as by generic nursing students, that practice in the acute-care setting is not perceived to be a desirable long-term career goal does not bode well for future availability of practitioners. Recommendations for change in the acute-care practice environment are clear. Such change might stem the flow of professional nurses away from this major practice site.

Sixteen percent of the senior RN/BSN students would like to be working in nursing administration in 10 years, and 15% would like to be working as clinical nurse specialists. More than half expect to continue working in the same nursing position in which they are currently employed.

These students were strongly inclined toward graduate education. By the end of the baccalaureate program, 70% indicated that they plan to pursue an advanced degree. This is congruent with the plans of generic students for postbaccalaureate education (Cassells et al., 1986b). As noted previously, 56.6% of students identify a desire to pursue a graduate degree as the original motivation for acquiring the bachelor's degree. The increase in the number of students identifying advanced education as a future career goal indicates a change in career goals and increased valuing of education as important to professional nursing. Thirteen percent of those indicating interest in continuing their education at the graduate level expected to enroll immediately; an additional 29%, in 2 to 11 months, and a group of 39%, within 1 to 2 years. Two thirds of the respondents felt they would need to attend school on a part-time basis. They would be dependent on personal earnings from employment and on personal savings as well as employer tuition reimbursement plans and scholarships/grants.

Nearly all of those indicating interest in graduate education in nursing expected to earn the master's degree; 14% were interested in obtaining a doctoral degree in nursing. Fourteen percent of the total sample indicated interest in a non-nursing advanced degree, with half choosing the field of business/management. This also is congruent with findings from generic baccalaureate students (Cassells et al., 1986b).

## SUMMARY

Transfer/challenge policies are best established in the liberal arts and sciences. The strongest concentration of clinical experience and faculty supervision is in community health/home care nursing. The type and quantity of clinical experiences reported by RN students warrant further investigation to clarify student responses in this study.

RN students are characteristically part-time students and full-time employees. The RN student works an average of 32 hours a week, a finding corroborated by other studies. As a result, average time for completion of the BSN program is 2 years with full-time attendance and 3.7 years with part-time attendance. But more important, completion rates reported for students admitted a decade earlier are high. This is a positive sign that students are being supported and are having their needs met.

In general, students' perceptions of their growth and their satisfaction with policies is strong. They report significant learning in nursing theories/models, geriatrics, public/community health, and nursing diagnosis. Unfortunately, many respondents reported difficulty with application of some of the content, notably theories/ models of nursing practice. This finding has implications for both the practice and the education communities.

Although many students expect to return to positions they are currently holding or have recently held, their long-term goals are strongly inclined toward graduate education and work in a variety of practice settings, more often away from the acute-care environment. Chapter 5 presents data on the postgraduation transition of these students.

## REFERENCES

American Association of Colleges of Nursing. (1986). *Essentials of college and university education for professional nursing.* Washington, DC: Author.

Arlton, D. M., & Miller, M. E. (1987). RN to BSN: Advanced placement policies. *Nurse Educator, 12*(6), 11–14.

Bednash, G., Redman, B., & Southers, N. (1989). *The economic investment in nursing education: Student, institutional, and clinical perspectives.* Washington, DC: Author.

Cassells, J. M., Redman, B. K., & Jackson, S. S. (1986a). Generic baccalaureate nursing student satisfaction regarding professional and personal development prior to graduation and one year postgraduation. *Journal of Professional Nursing, 2,* 114–127.

Cassells, J. M., Redman, B. K., & Jackson, S. S. (1986b). Student choice of baccalaureate nursing programs, their perceived level of growth and development, career plans, and transition into practice. *Journal of Professional Nursing, 2,* 186–196.

Council on Postsecondary Accreditation & American Association of Collegiate Registrars and Admissions Officers. (1979). *Joint statement on transfer and award of academic credit.* Washington, DC: Author.

National League for Nursing. (1987). *Methods for awarding credit for previously acquired nursing knowledge and competency.* New York: Author.

Shane, D. L. (1983). *Returning to school: A guide for nurses.* Englewood Cliffs, NJ: Prentice-Hall.

Woolley, A. S. (1984). The bridge course: transition to professional practice. *Nurse Educator, 9*(4), 15–19.

# 5

# Transition Back into the Work Environment

Transition back into the workplace can be viewed through several lenses, one of which is reviewing published information about psychosocial adaptation to the transition back to work. From the RN Baccalaureate Nursing Education Data Project, data were gathered 6 months postgraduation about advancement in the job marketplace and about graduates' estimates of their level of skill and application of what was learned during the BSN program and of their progress toward graduate education.

Just as the transition to school was described in the context of the returning-to-school syndrome (Shane, 1983), so transition back to the workplace can present a kind of reentry shock. The workplace does not necessarily change during the RN student's education. Because some educationally mobile nurses may return to school as a way of dealing with burnout, facing those old concerns precipitates frustration and anger. In addition, one nurse reflected that if schools of nursing truly taught one how to handle problematic issues in nursing—such as the wide differences between theory and clinical practice, the shortage of good nurses, low salaries, tremendous job responsibilities, and poor hours—perhaps returning RNs would have a set of strategies that would help them cope after graduation (Shane, Dixson, & Moldenhauer, 1983). But the goals of the baccalaureate are not uniquely or perhaps even squarely focused on these issues.

## DEMOGRAPHICS AND CURRENT JOB
## SITUATIONS OF GRADUATES

Fully 94% of RN/BSN graduates reported being currently employed as RNs, three fourths of them full-time. Fifty-seven percent were working in the same job they held prior to completing the BSN, and nearly 75% of that group reported that the bachelor's degree was not necessary to obtain or maintain their current RN positions. Of the 42% who were not working in the same position, more than half had changed employers. Of these, 27% reported that a bachelor's degree was necessary to obtain or maintain their current RN position.

Most (83%) were employed in the same geographic setting, defined as within 50 miles of where they went to school to obtain the bachelor's degree. Despite the strong focus on community and home health in the baccalaureate program, nearly 80% of these graduates were working in hospitals, 3% each in community/public health nursing and home health nursing and 3% in nursing homes. Two thirds indicated they were working in their desired nursing positions. Of 318 (74%) RN graduates working in hospitals, 28% worked in hospitals with 100–299 beds, 33% in hospitals with 300–449 beds, and 32% in hospitals with 500 or more beds. About 6% were employed in hospitals with fewer than 100 beds.

Within hospitals, RN graduates worked most frequently in medical-surgical units (14.1%), emergency rooms (14.1%), critical care units (12.8%), obstetrics (8.4%), and psychiatric/mental health units (5.5%). More than 12% of the RN graduates reported working in multiple areas in a supervisory or float capacity.

As is true generally in the nursing marketplace, more than 70% of these RN/BSN graduates had not received a pay differential, at the time the study was conducted, for having earned the degree. If such a differential was given, it averaged 5.8%, or an additional $1,300. Also, there was no significant difference for the cohort in the profile of jobs they held before and after receiving the baccalaureate. The 6-month follow-up was perhaps too short a time to note eventual differences.

Senior RN students rated the relative importance of factors in a nursing position as they recalled their preferences prior to entering

**TABLE 5.1. RN Students' Perceptions of Importance of Factors in an RN Position ($n = 742$)**

| Factor | No. | Prior to program | | Completion of program | | t | p |
|---|---|---|---|---|---|---|---|
| | | Mean[a] | SD | Mean[a] | SD | | |
| Opportunity to participate in policymaking | 709 | 4.13 | 1.42 | 5.35 | .90 | −24.68 | <.001 |
| Philosophy of institution complements personal/professional philosophy | 709 | 3.97 | 1.57 | 5.18 | 1.03 | −22.69 | <.001 |
| Opportunity for advancement | 705 | 4.80 | 1.19 | 5.70 | .65 | −21.28 | <.001 |
| Good communication channels | 708 | 4.89 | 1.19 | 5.70 | .62 | −20.27 | <.001 |
| Opportunity to work as a peer with other health team members | 711 | 4.78 | 1.19 | 5.59 | .68 | −19.79 | <.001 |
| Organization of patient care | 709 | 4.20 | 1.41 | 5.07 | 1.16 | −19.77 | <.001 |
| Opportunity to work to full potential | 709 | 4.98 | 1.19 | 5.73 | .61 | −19.02 | <.001 |
| Opportunities for professional growth | 712 | 4.85 | 1.19 | 5.66 | .72 | −18.60 | <.001 |
| Support from supervisory personnel | 708 | 4.94 | 1.20 | 5.64 | .71 | −17.09 | <.001 |
| Adequate staffing | 707 | 5.11 | 1.13 | 5.70 | .66 | −15.61 | <.001 |
| Working environment | 708 | 5.23 | 1.00 | 5.74 | .58 | −15.09 | <.001 |

**TABLE 5.1.** (continued)

| Factor | No. | Prior to program Mean[a] | SD | Completion of program Mean[a] | SD | $t$ | $p$ |
|---|---|---|---|---|---|---|---|
| Salary | 706 | 5.11 | 1.03 | 5.59 | .67 | −14.5 | <.001 |
| Preceptor/nurse internship program | 684 | 4.08 | 1.61 | 4.78 | 1.48 | −14.02 | <.001 |
| Adequate length of time for orientation | 708 | 4.89 | 1.19 | 5.45 | .86 | −13.54 | <.001 |
| Hours and shifts | 707 | 5.16 | 1.13 | 5.64 | .77 | −12.80 | <.001 |
| Benefits | 709 | 5.10 | 1.09 | 5.55 | .76 | −12.39 | <.001 |
| Type of patient care setting | 707 | 4.96 | 1.15 | 5.36 | .91 | −12.06 | <.001 |
| Type of patients admitted | 705 | 4.26 | 1.49 | 4.58 | 1.45 | −9.76 | <.001 |
| Geographic location of institution | 712 | 5.04 | 1.21 | 5.12 | 1.11 | −2.42 | .016 |

[a]1, very unimportant; 2, moderately unimportant; 3, slightly unimportant; 4, slightly important; 5, moderately important; 6, very important.

the BSN program and at the time of data collection in their senior year; these data are shown in Table 5.1. Although importance ratings prior to the program generally reflect what is known about these factors, the fascinating finding is the change in perceived importance at the close of the program. All factors showed significant change in level of importance, but some of the greatest changes can be seen in the following: "Philosophy of the institution complements personal/professional philosophy," "Opportunity to participate in policymaking," "Opportunity to work as a peer with other

**TABE 5.2. Level of Satisfaction with Job-Related Factors in Current Positions, 6-Months Postgraduation ($n = 427$)**

| Factor | No. | Mean[a] | SD |
|---|---|---|---|
| Quality of care provided at institution | 404 | 3.27 | .81 |
| Opportunity to work as a peer with other health team members | 402 | 3.18 | .83 |
| Philosophy of institution complements personal/professional philosophy | 410 | 3.06 | .82 |
| Organization of nursing care, primary care nursing | 287 | 2.99 | .91 |
| Fringe benefits | 388 | 2.95 | .90 |
| Support from supervisory personnel | 412 | 2.92 | .96 |
| Opportunity to work to full potential | 412 | 2.88 | 1.02 |
| Opportunity to participate in decision making | 411 | 2.82 | .98 |
| Orientation program | 403 | 2.81 | .93 |
| Continuing education/inservice programs | 402 | 2.79 | .94 |
| Communication channels | 411 | 2.75 | .96 |
| Retirement plans | 378 | 2.68 | .97 |
| Salary and compensation | 409 | 2.67 | .91 |
| Organization of nursing care, team nursing | 191 | 2.64 | .92 |
| Staffing patterns | 397 | 2.58 | .94 |
| Tuition-reimbursement program for master's | 336 | 2.53 | 1.10 |
| Opportunity for promotion and advancement | 398 | 2.51 | 1.01 |

[a]1, not satisfied; 2, minimally satisfied; 3, satisfied; 4, very satisfied.

health team members," "advancement," and "Opportunities for professional growth." These changes are consistent with further socialization to a professional role.

The actual level of satisfaction of the new RN/BSN graduates at 6 months is presented in Table 5.2. On the average, many factors clustered slightly above and below "satisfied." "Staffing patterns," "Tuition-reimbursement program for master's" and "Opportunity for promotion and advancement" were least satisfactory. Several of the factors that showed a significant increase in importance over the course of the baccalaureate program were rated in excess of satisfactory ("Opportunity to work as a peer with other health team members" and "Philosophy of institution complements personal/ professional philosophy); others were less satisfactory ("Opportunity for promotion and advancement" and "Communication channels").

## GRADUATES' ESTIMATES OF SKILL LEVELS AND IMPORTANCE OF CONTENT TO CLINICAL PRACTICE

In general, the individuals studied gave estimates of the importance of coursework to clinical nursing practice and of their own skills in nursing subject matter that were similar at 6 months postgraduation to those given at the time of graduation.

An effort was made to determine whether the kinds of patient care decisions/activities of these new graduates had changed, compared with their functions prior to earning the BSN. On items such as discharge planning, responsibility for primary care, serving as team leader, being member of a quality assurance committee, there were no differences. More of the graduates indicated they were members of nursing practice standards committees than had been the case pre-BSN.

Perhaps these findings were to be expected because, for the most part, RN positions are not differentiated by educational preparation. A few institutions are establishing systems of differentiated practice, in which nurses perform distinct jobs (technical or professional) based on their educational preparation. The factors cited as driving forces toward differentiation of practice into professional and technical roles are the complexity of health care needs of patients; the shift of health care services to settings outside the hospital, where nurses must function independently; and the continuation of rapid change in health care settings, services, and technology (NCNIP, 1987).

## PROGRESS TOWARD GRADUATE EDUCATION

Near the time of completion of their baccalaureate education, 72% of students indicated an interest in obtaining a graduate degree. Thirteen percent of those indicating interest expected to enroll immediately, with an additional 29% within 2 to 11 months. At 6-months postgraduation, 17% of those responding to the follow-up survey indicated that they were enrolled full-time or part-time in a graduate program, with an additional 7% indicating that they had applied to a program to begin soon. This is a faster move into graduate education than was found among new generic baccalaureate graduates: 4% were pursuing an advanced degree at a similar time of follow-up (Cassells, Redman, & Jackson, 1986b). Only 22% of the RN/BSN follow-up respondents indicated they were not intending to pursue advanced/graduate education.

The group saw the master's degree as the immediate goal, with only 8% indicating any interest in doctoral education. Certification in a nursing specialty was of interest to one fifth of respondents; usually preparation for certification occurs during the master's program. Sources of financial support for pursuing graduate education were most commonly personal savings, earnings from employment, and employer tuition-reimbursement plans. Twenty-nine percent of those enrolled in master's-degree programs were in non-nursing fields; this proportion is identical to that found in the study of generic baccalaureate graduates (Cassells, Redman, & Jackson, 1986a).

It would seem clear that the master's degree is the real goal for a significant portion of RN students. Greater than 56% of RN students identified the master's degree as a significant pre-enrollment motivator for acquiring the bachelor's degree. By the end of the program, 70% of the students wished to achieve the master's de-

gree. And following graduation, almost 80% of respondents identified the master's degree as either an immediate or future goal.
Indeed, there is considerable interest among schools in creating
RN-MSN programs, capitalizing on this motivation. Creative RN-
MSN educational opportunities could greatly facilitate the acquisition of advanced education for large numbers of registered nurses.
However, the expressed dissatisfaction with the availability of
tuition-reimbursement programs for support of the nurse acquiring
the master's degree highlights the need to expand available tuition
support programs and to identify for employers the benefits of
supporting the employee who seeks the advanced degree.

Finally, some believe that professionalism can be measured in
part by membership in one's professional organizations. Thirty percent of follow-up respondents report being members of the American Nurses' Association, a rate considerably higher than for the
general population of RNs. Nearly an equal number report membership in a specialty nursing society.

## SUMMARY

Previous work, primarily anecdotal in nature, describes a sometimes
painful reentry transition into the workplace for new RN/BSN graduates. In the present study, nearly all new RN/BSN graduates returned to the workplace, more than half of them in the same job.
However, most of them received no additional pay for having the
degree and were working in positions that did not require it. The
failure of employers to differentiate the practice environment requirements and the lack of compensation for the employee who
brings enhanced skills and knowledge to the nursing position have
been identified as critical concerns in the present nursing shortage.
The Secretary's Commission on Nursing (USDHHS, 1988) has recommended the following:

> Health care delivery organizations should adopt innovative nurse staff-
> ing patterns that recognize and appropriately utilize the different lev-
> els of education, competence, and experience among registered
> nurses. . . . Additionally, they should pursue the development and
> implementation of innovative compensation options for nurses and

expand pay-ranges based on experience, performance, education, and demonstrated leadership. (pp. vi, vii)

It is instructive, or should be, that large numbers of these students report a desire to leave the acute-care setting. Perhaps the failure of this practice environment to adequately recognize, through compensation or work responsibilities, the additional resources the nurse brings to the service environment after completing the BS degree is a factor in this apparent flight from a major practice environment.

The large number of nurses pursuing graduate degrees in nursing is a positive sign for the future of professional nursing. This nation sorely needs expert nurse clinicians, administrators, and researchers. The data show that graduate education was the real goal for many of these new graduates.

## REFERENCES

Cassells, J. M., Redman, B. K., & Jackson, S. S. (1986a). Generic baccalaureate nursing student satisfaction regarding professional and personal development prior to graduation and one year postgraduation. *Journal of Professional Nursing*, 2, 114–127.

Cassells, J. M., Redman, B. K., & Jackson, S. S. (1986b). Student choice of baccalaureate nursing programs, their perceived level of growth and development, career plans, and transition into practice: A replication. *Journal of Professional Nursing*, 2, 186–196.

National Commission on Nursing Implementation Project. (1987). A progress report on differentiated practice. Milwaukee, WI: Author.

Shane, D. L. (1983). *Returning to school: A guide for nurses.* Englewood Cliffs, NJ: Prentice-Hall.

Shane, D. L., Dixson, J., & Moldenhauer, M. (1983). Back to work: More transitions? In D. L. Shane, (Ed.), *Returning to school: A guide for nurses.* Englewood Cliffs, NJ: Prentice-Hall.

U.S. Department of Health and Human Services, Secretary's Commission on Nursing. (1988). *Final report.* Washington, DC: Author.

# 6

# Summary and Policy
# Implications of the
# AACN Study

This chapter summarizes the AACN study through reviewing questions raised earlier in the book: What is the nature of the "movement" of RNs returning to obtain the BSN? The degree of access for RNs to BSN education? The speed with which they progress through the program? The nature of the education they undergo and their satisfaction with it? And how are their newly learned skills utilized in the workplace? We also will put the findings into a broader policy-based perspective.

A summary of the major findings of the study follows:

• It would seem that we have entered a fourth era of RN/BSN education, one of greatly widened access. BSN education for RNs is now considerably more accessible than is BSN education for generic students. Virtually all programs that accept generic students also accept RN students, and more than 100 schools admit *only* RNs to their BSN programs. Students report no wait for admission. Evening, year-round, and part-time study options are widely available, as are satellite/outreach locations for instruction, and they are being used by students. In addition, 61% of programs report plans to expand their capacity for RN/BSN education, thus probably increasing access.

• Besides their interest in personal growth, students seem to have been motivated to enter the BSN program by signals they were getting from the marketplace and by their interest in graduate education. In fact, the motivation to pursue an advanced degree was a significant preenrollment and postgraduation goal for future career growth. At 6 months after graduation, 17% of respondents indicated they were enrolled in graduate study. Perhaps the most important outcomes of the BSN program for these students is their strong perceived preparation for graduate education and their confidence in their academic abilities and in their general academic knowledge.

• The RN student is characteristically a part-time student who engages in studies around the life responsibilities already acquired prior to baccalaureate studies. A large percentage of the RN/BSN students report that they are employed full-time during their studies. These students therefore require a longer time period in which to complete the bachelor's degree. On the average, their programs were completed in 2 years if they attended full-time and in 3.7 years if they attended part-time; and deans indicated that within a span of 10 years, nearly 90% had completed the degree.

• Transfer of previous credit is common in the basic sciences, especially in microbiology, psychology, sociology, and anatomy/ physiology. Nursing coursework is more often likely to be challengeable, although one quarter of the schools report accepting credits for these areas by transfer. Students were generally satisfied with their programs and in all areas perceived significant growth from beginning to end of the program.

• The new BSN graduates returned overwhelmingly to nursing employment in hospitals in the same geographic setting in which they went to school. They reported being in positions that did not require the bachelor's degree and receiving no pay increase for having achieved it. However, their perceptions of desirable factors in the work setting—for example, congruence of the institution with their own professional philosophy, opportunity to participate in policymaking, opportunity to work as a peer with other health team members, good communication channels, and opportunity for advancement—increasingly reflect the importance of professionalism.

Several areas should receive additional study and attention:

• Both generic and RN students have rated their computer skills as poorly developed. They also report low levels of application of their knowledge in this area, perhaps in part because work settings are not highly computerized. Students reported moderate levels of use of theories/models of nursing in their clinical practice, which also should be further studied. Certainly, the recently released final report of the Secretary's Commission on Nursing (US-DHHS, 1988) emphasized the need to increase computerization of the nursing work environment to facilitate the proper use of nursing skills or knowledge. It appears that both the educational environment and the practice environment need to address more effectively issues of computerization of nursing work.

• This study did not provide in-depth understanding of the nature of clinical experience for RN students, especially with patterns of successful challenge of clinical nursing courses. A significant number of RN students reported that they did not engage in clinical experience as part of acquiring the bachelors' degree. This is a significant finding and requires further explication to determine its accuracy and its implications for professional nursing development.

• Although many individuals change fields of study at the graduate level, the fact that 29% of new RN/BSN graduates enrolled in master's-degree programs in non-nursing fields is cause for further follow-up study. A large number of this group chose study in management, even though many schools of nursing offer majors in nursing administration at the master's level. The American Association of Colleges of Nursing and the American Organization of Nurse Executives (1986) have taken the position that since the nurse executives are responsible for leadership and management of the nursing organization and accountable for the clinical practice of nursing, as well as functioning as members of the executive management team, their educational preparation should take place in collegiate schools of nursing offering specialized graduate programs in nursing management.

## IS THERE A MOVEMENT?

It would indeed seem that a movement is occurring in the large-scale return of RNs to obtain the BSN, despite the lack of obvious short-term benefits of having earned the degree. To an extraordinary extent, the system of nursing education has promoted, assisted in, and accommodated this movement. Clearly, nurse educators have been tremendously responsive to the issues of access and flexibility in providing opportunity for RNs to return to acquire the bachelor's degree. The tremendous increase in the use of satellite/ outreach programs, alternative scheduling, transfer of credits, and so on, identifies the interest nurse educators have in facilitating the movement of RNs toward the bachelor's degree.

The issue that continually gets confused with this large-scale return to school is whether the entire system of nursing education should be restructured to make the two-stage preparation for the BSN norm. Despite the fact that an entire sector of nursing education has grown up to meet the need for the second step and the fact that some states have legislation that is intended to protect the currency of previous education and experience for RNs, there are several forces working against such a conversion of the educational system.

The force that has not been clearly recognized is that the system of higher education in general has only a partially developed structure for transfer/challenge from one level to another. This means that if nursing were to have a predominantly two-level structure, not only would it be out of the mainstream of higher education, but in the absence of a broader system of transfer agreements, schools would continue to have to develop ad hoc approaches to dealing with previous credit and experience. There are, of course, also questions of the additional cost for such a system, although precise, widely generalizable data on this question do not seem to be available. However, it is clear that attempts to provide flexibility and access require additional resources (i.e., increased costs) as the nursing program attempts to respond to the diverse needs of the returning student.

Another force that mitigates against a move to a permanent 2 + 2 system is that organized nursing needs to recruit individuals from a variety of life circumstances and educational backgrounds. In addition, the profession is intent on further development and promotion of the professional level of practice, stemming in large part from the conviction that nursing care needs of the public require wide availability of individuals with a higher level of preparation.

Already the profession has to deal with the disincentives in the marketplace for investing in the BSN. The failure of the practice environment to focus on educational preparation as a basis for professional practice could be further confused by widespread use of a two-tiered system. In addition, previous studies have shown that two thirds of generic baccalaureate nursing students never considered an ADN or diploma nursing program and that a significant part of their motivation is to obtain a college degree. One would have to wonder whether such individuals would be lost to the profession in a 2 + 2 system. Certainly, individuals who prefer the traditional bachelor's degree process would likely be unwilling to first enroll in an associate degree program prior to being allowed access to the baccalaureate program.

In reality, nursing has adapted to the need to upgrade the RN population in a way that is characteristic of the higher education system in this country—through diverse and multiple approaches. In fact, the adaptation and responsiveness of the RN/BSN programs is evidence of nurse educators' commitment to the need for a highly educated cadre of professional nurses. It is likely that multiple options will continue to exist, affected in part by the availability of generic students and by changes in licensing laws, externally mandated educational options, and incentives in the workplace.

The authors have informal information that schools that started as RN-only programs are considering making the transition to admitting generic students, just as most generic programs have now moved to admit RN students and are more rapidly exploring segments for RN/BSN education. Taking advantage of the drive of some RN students to obtain the master's degree, some schools have initiated RN/MSN programs. Both of these moves provide further evidence of the need to make available the BS and MS as preferred routes and levels of preparation.

## OTHER ISSUES

The study has raised several other issues that are worth pursuing because they might improve the efficiency and effectiveness of the system. The lack of a standardized set of outcomes from the baccalaureate curriculum has meant that transfer anywhere within the nursing education system has been more difficult. Two national commissions, completing their work in 1983, concluded that (1) the nursing profession must outline the common body of knowledge and skills essential for nursing practice, the curriculum content that supports it, and a credentialing process that reinforces it (National Commission on Nursing, 1983); and (2) the lack of consensus on objectives and performance measures for graduates of different types of nursing education programs creates problems for nursing education and for nursing service (Institute of Medicine, 1983). The *Essentials* were the result of a broad consensus-building and consensus-testing process (AACN, 1986). This document represents the profession's definition of essential elements of preparation for professional nursing and, along with formalized tools measuring accomplishment of the elements, could form a structure for easier verification and transfer of credit.

A second question relates to systems for ensuring quality in educational programs. Because about half of the RN-only programs do not fall under the jurisdiction of the state board of nursing, and National League for Nursing accreditation is voluntary, it is likely that a portion of these schools have not undergone any discipline-based accreditation process. This is true for 16% of respondent schools.

## PREDICTION FOR THE FUTURE

The adjustment of BSN programs to RN students has been incremental since the early part of this century. Several characteristics of the higher education system in this country have affected this evolution. The system is one of the most market-oriented in the world (Clark, 1983) and has probably responded more vigorously in recent years to the RN/BSN market because of the decline in both the number of traditional students and the number interested in nursing. The system also responds to organized special interest groups. Not only have potential RN/BSN students organized to press their special interests, but community and junior colleges, which provided 41,300 ADN graduates in 1985–86 (NLN, 1988), also have a large stake in a system that provides articulation made as easy as possible. The fact that some ADN programs require in excess of 100 semester hours for completion, whereas baccalaureate programs currently require 130 semester hours, means that RN students have a bigger stake in transfer and articulation policies than they would have if the credit requirements for the two degrees were more carefully balanced.

These forces can be expected to continue to exert pressure on BSN programs. And as enrollment in diploma programs continues to decline dramatically, it is possible that the system of RN/BSN education will become more standardized to the needs of the ADN graduate. In addition, diploma-prepared nurses have shown a greater indication to obtain the BSN and higher degrees (16%) than have ADN graduates (10%) (ANA, 1987), and the shift to a greater percentage of nurses who are ADN-prepared may signal a decline in RN/BSN enrollment. But much more basic changes may be in store if the single RN license is altered to create different licenses for technical and professional practitioners and the workplace makes more distinct differentiations between the roles. The relative pay scales and role responsibilities of these two categories of nurse will likely create less or more demand for RN/BSN education.

As all of higher education serves increasingly diverse groups of students, the field must become adept at processes of inclusion. The experience with RNs would suggest that (1) a database be established to provide accurate information about access to education for the new groups; (2) replicable models of good quality that can be adapted to local conditions be well publicized; (3) advisory groups be established at all levels of the profession to ensure good communication and problem solving; (4) a clash of cultures must be expected; and (5) resources, including tests, will be necessary and made available to establish the integrative mechanisms.

The movement of RN students to obtain the BSN is indeed a movement, and a significant one. Through the actions of many individuals, it signals a strong consensus about the necessity of this preparation in contemporary nursing practice and the importance of appropriate education for the professional role. The movement is a laudable accomplishment for the profession. It represents both a philosophy and a structure through which individuals can upgrade their skills and by which the profession itself can become more cohesive.

## REFERENCES

American Association of Colleges of Nursing. (1986). *Essentials of college and university education for professional nursing.* Washington, DC: Author.

American Association of Colleges of Nursing & American Organization of Nurse Executives. (1986). Position statement on graduate education in nursing administration. *Journal of Professional Nursing, 2,* 263.

American Nurses' Association. (1987). *Facts about nursing, 1986–87.* Kansas City, MO: Author.

Clark, B. (1983). *The higher education system.* Berkeley, CA: University of California Press.

Institute of Medicine. (1983). *Nursing and nursing education: Public policies and private actions.* Washington, DC: National Academy Press.

Iowa Board of Nursing. (1988). *A statewide plan for nursing.* Des Moines, IA: Author.

National Commission on Nursing. (1983). *Summary report and recommendations.* Chicago: Author.

National League for Nursing. (1988). *Nursing data review 1987.* New York: Author.

U. S. Department of Health and Human Services, Secretary's Commission on Nursing. (1988). *Final report.* Washington, DC: Author.

# 7
# The Baccalaureate Menu:
# Different Educational Models

## Alma S. Woolley, Ed.D., R.N.

Registered nurses prepared in associate degree or diploma programs have many choices to make when planning their educational pathways toward bachelor's and higher degrees. According to the data on which this book is based, only 3% of all baccalaureate programs do not admit RNs at all and many baccalaureate programs are for RNs only; therefore, the RN has a much wider choice of programs than the generic student has.

Various curriculum models are outlined in Table 2.2 (Chapter 2). Lack of unanimity about the most effective way to offer the professional degree to RNs is the result of more than regional or economic factors. Indeed, most of the issues that arise in any discussion of this kind of education have their roots in differing nursing education philosophies.

## TECHNICAL VERSUS PROFESSIONAL: A CONTINUING DEBATE

The major issue on which consensus is still lacking is the relationship between technical and professional nursing. The difference was very clear to Montag (cited in Kelly, 1985) when she coordinated a demonstration project at Teachers' College, Columbia University, in 1952; she saw no problem in preparing a nurse with some general education, whose expertise would lie in giving direct care to persons with common nursing problems, who would be directed and supervised by other personnel, and who would see this limited scope of practice as a long-term occupation.

The designation "professional" was to be reserved for nurses with the minimum of a baccalaureate. Their programs were to be designed from the beginning to prepare them to deal with a much larger scope of specific as well as general nursing problems, to use nursing theory to guide and shape practice, and to lead and manage other personnel (including technical nurses), not only as a result of different content in the baccalaureate program but because of the influence of the liberal arts and humanities courses that were essential components of this curriculum.

This concept was, however, never really accepted by the majority of nurses or even nurse educators. Instructors in associate degree programs, most with bachelor's and master's degrees, continued to teach nursing as they themselves knew it and practiced it. Nurses who had passed their state board examinations continued to call themselves professional nurses, as many were designated on their licenses.

Diploma education found itself in a kind of limbo. Once the bastion of professionalism, these hospital-sponsored schools resisted being categorized as technical merely because they did not confer the baccalaureate. Many kept pace with curriculum developments by choosing particular nursing theories, adding research and community health components, and bringing their student rules and regulations into line with collegiate programs. Faculty qualifications were raised and additional non-nursing courses required as part of their programs.

In 1974 and again in 1988, members of the Council of Associate Degree Programs of the National League for Nursing rejected the descriptor "technical" for their programs or their graduates. Baccalaureate educators have, however, persisted in using the offensive term to describe both associate degree and diploma graduates. The National Commission on Nursing Implementation Project (NCNIP) continues to use "technical" and "professional" preparation to describe the two categories of nurses who will be in place by 2010 (see Chapter 1, Appendix).

The philosophical basis of all of this semantic disagreement is the relationship of the content and terminal objectives of the two (or three) kinds of nursing education programs, which Montag (Kelly, 1985) saw as very different. Those who still accept her premise use the analogy of dental assistants to dentistry; one does not precede the other (Fig. 7.1). According to Martha Rogers (1964),

> Registered nurses, who have prepared for a technical career in nursing through completion of an associate degree or hospital school program of study, and who later decide they wish to prepare for a professional career in nursing, will have had *no* courses in nursing equivalent to baccalaureate degree courses in the professional nursing major. Nor will they, in either case, have had the prerequisites to comprehend upper division nursing science courses. Technical education is complete in itself.

The implication of this belief is that a person wishing to change career direction would need to begin again at the beginning, and some of the baccalaureate programs in the middle era discussed in Chapter 1 were based on this assumption. They did not use the terms "degree completion" or even "second step" because they believed that technical nursing education could not be considered a predecessor to the professional level.

Another implication of this belief that held sway during the 1970s was that baccalaureate graduates need not be "technically"

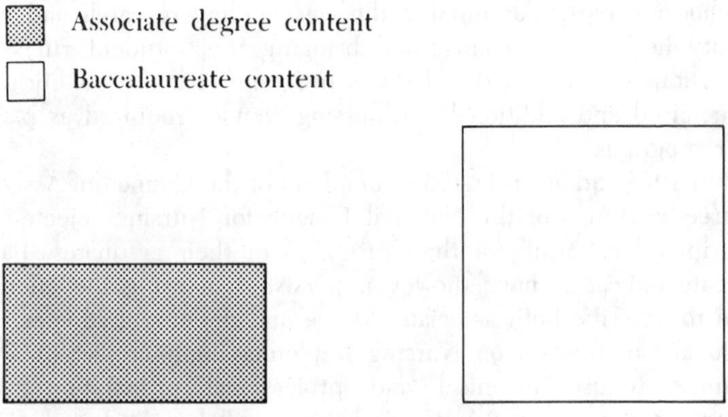

Associate degree content

Baccalaureate content

**Figure 7.1.** Two separate bodies of content

proficient as long as they could use the nursing process appropriately. "The philosophy and purposes of professional education are ill-served by emphasis on specific skills. A properly educated worker will pick up proficiency in 'how-to-do-it' in a minimum of time" (Rogers, 1964). The task of seeing that graduates could perform the skills necessary to implement the care plans was delegated to, but not cheerfully acccepted by, the initial employer, who resented the additional expense involved in a prolonged orientation period for these nurses.

## TESTING/CHALLENGING/VALIDATING

The concept of a "terminal degree" also turned out to be just too un-American, as well as antithetic to the egalitarian climate of nursing. Many baccalaureate programs attempted to isolate the portions of content that were common to both programs and to develop mechanisms for validating mastery of these portions by technical nurses (Fig. 7.2). This concept can also be represented as two concentric circles, with the larger, or professional, encompassing the smaller, or technical, core.

Each program, being somewhat different from every other pro-

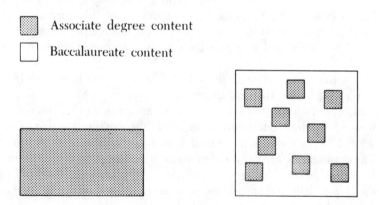

□ Associate degree content

□ Baccalaureate content

**Figure 7.2.** Content of one contained in other

gram, felt justified in requiring specific teacher-made or course-end tests to be passed in order to exempt the RN students from courses or portions of courses (Rogers, 1976). This testing activity often became an overwhelming task for faculty members and a source of resentment on the part of practicing nurses, who did not understand the need for validating what they were already doing.

Validation of clinical competency became another hurdle for both faculty and potential students. Written tests could validate knowledge, but how could faculty members be assured that students who had graduated from another type of program could fulfill the clinical objectives of the course? Should the students who challenged the content of a medical-surgical nursing course demonstrate technical practice (which they had already learned) or professional practice (which they had not yet learned) in the clinical area? Elaborate and time-consuming mechanisms were set up to test clinical competence so that faculty could be assured that each RN student could give care at the same level as the basic students in the program. The potential for conflict and anger was built into this process, especially when nurses who had been practicing for many years were being tested. A statement from the NLN Council of Baccalaureate and Higher Degree Programs in 1982 strongly urged that this testing be done.

Since many schools have devised various strategies to circumvent this procedure, and others simply ignore it, the revised accreditation criteria (NLN, 1988) do not specify that this clinical testing must be done. Instead, schools will need to carefully demonstrate the consistency and rationale for whatever testing procedures they choose.

A third conception of the relationship between these two levels of nursing is one that is diametrically opposed to Montag's original idea (Fig. 7.3). In this version, the American dream of onward and upward through education is realized: the technical nurse simply adds 2 years on to her original 2 and emerges as a professional. These programs carefully differentiate which portion of the curriculum they believe belongs at each level; the student "tests out" of the lower half and takes the complete upper half in a specially designed program "for RNs only."

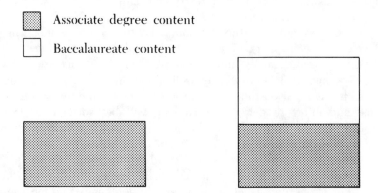

**Figure 7.3.** Baccalaureate builds on associate degree

## MAKING THE TRANSITION

The differences between technically and professionally prepared nurses are believed to extend beyond the curriculum to one's whole perspective on nursing and health care. Some of the distance between these differences can be closed by the generous addition of liberal arts and humanities courses to the education of the technical nurse, but most educators agree that a satisfactory metamorphosis requires two other ingredients: a "bridge" course and exposure time.

The bridge course is usually the first course in the nursing curriculum and is designed to facilitate students' transition from the technical to the professional level of practice. Its purpose is to thoroughly orient them to the philosophy of the curriculum they will be pursuing and to demonstrate the necessity of the "conscious, continual application of theory to practice" (Woolley, 1984). By the end of the course, students should have a clear idea of the conceptual framework of the program and of what the rest of the curriculum will consist. Concepts that do not receive much attention on the associate degree level can be expanded—for example, stress, change, loss and grief, pain, poverty and deprivation, and a review of the whole spectrum of nursing theories.

The RNs entering the program take the course alone. They develop a peer support group to help them deal with the inevitable pressures from families and fellow workers. The success of the whole educational venture may well hinge on this experience because it often assists students in deciding whether the investment of time and effort to get a baccalaureate will be worthwhile. It is crucial that this course be taught by faculty members with a thorough understanding of and commitment to its objectives, as well as an understanding of the principles of adult education.

Exposure time is also believed to be crucial in effecting the transition from one level to another. Students need to be with faculty and other professional practitioners for a long enough period for them to understand and assimilate the differences between the level of practice they have learned and the level they are expected to attain. In recent years, the movement to accelerate the educational process has meant less emphasis on this factor and may result in increased blurring of roles of graduates.

## TRANSFER OF CREDIT

Of major importance to all RNs considering earning a baccalaureate is the number of credits they are granted by their educational institution for the courses they have taken elsewhere; this is a major determiner of how long the next step in their education will take. The most common practice in the early and middle periods of RN-to-BSN education was to accept only transfer of non-nursing courses, and then only when each specific course was approved by the comparable department in the university. As a result, many RNs repeated such courses as chemistry, anatomy, and physiology because their original courses were not approved. In the past decade, there has been a move to accept almost any comparable non-nursing course without individual evaluation because exact matches of content are almost impossible.

Nursing programs have been less flexible in accepting nursing courses. Because diploma school courses carry no academic credit, they are rarely accepted. Instead, the applicant takes challenge exams to receive credit and advanced placement in the baccalaureate curriculum.

Associate degree courses do carry academic credit. However, most baccalaureate programs accept the model depicted in Figure 7.2 as representing the relationship between the content of the two kinds of programs; therefore, they have been reluctant to transfer courses as a whole, and they also require associate degree graduates to take challenge exams.

Some states, such as Maryland, have successfully mandated the transfer of all courses completed at approved community colleges since 1979 to the state university system. Students who graduated prior to 1979 have the choice of taking advanced placement examinations or three transition courses that carry equivalent lower-division credit (Rapson, 1987). The first reported study of this articulation scheme showed that there was no difference in the academic achievement of 113 students admitted via these three pathways.

Hospital diploma schools, still caught between the two levels, continue to fight for survival. Many have closed because of lack of applicants and escalating expenses. Others have made alliances with community colleges so that their nursing courses are given credit toward an associate degree in science. Others have revised their curricula and affiliated with 4-year colleges to offer the baccalaureate. Most of those remaining provide transferable non-nursing courses through community colleges and encourage their graduates to plan to go on for a degree later in their nursing careers.

## DIFFERENTIATION OF COMPETENCIES

One of the major obstacles to facilitating smooth transition from associate-degree or diploma education to the baccalaureate curriculum is the lack of agreement among these programs about the specific functions for which their graduates are prepared. Although several major studies have attempted to differentiate these competencies, the lack of implementation of this difference in job descriptions for graduates of each type of program, thereby necessitating separate licensure, is an impediment to devising a clear means of moving from one level to another.

## COMPARISON OF CURRICULUM MODELS

At least six different models for career mobility are currently in existence. The creativity of nurse educators, as well as economic incentives and exigencies, portend the appearance of several more. Each has its advocates and each needs to be understood and considered by the RN contemplating entering a baccalaureate program.

### Integration into a Generic Program

Integration of the RN into the generic 4-year program was the original pattern of the middle era. The RN transfers as many non-nursing courses as fit into the curriculum, and then, based on the model shown in Figure 7.2, challenges nursing courses or parts of courses and takes whatever additional courses are necessary to qualify for the degree. All of the pieces are assembled into a baccalaureate that appears to contain the same content as the generic student has covered. The testing costs are usually borne by the student, and the program does not have to offer special courses or employ special faculty other than perhaps a counselor or coordinator to assist students through the maze.

Students in this model frequently do not agree that they are learning new material and complain of duplication. They dislike being in classes with young students. Instructors find the heterogeneity of the class difficult, particularly in the clinical area. Since all graduates are to achieve the same objectives, there may be some discomfort in allowing the RN students to do different or more advanced activities.

### Separate Track Within Generic Program

A modification of this pattern has been made in many programs by faculty who believe that they are able to sort out more clearly which part of the curriculum RNs have already mastered and which parts they need. A battery of "mobility tests" is used to measure achievement of a body of content, and certain courses in the curriculum (at the school's discretion) are considered validated if the student achieves the score designated by the school. RNs in these programs may be in a separate track in which their courses are primarily research, community health, and some form of leadership/ management experience along with the generic students.

These programs are closer to the model in Figure 7.3 in that they acknowledge a body of content that can be assumed to be present in both programs. Such programs usually provide also for a bridge course in which the RNs are oriented to baccalaureate philosophy and find their support group to see them through the rest of the program. Again, however, the terminal objectives of the program must be the same for both generic and RN students, and faculty members must find different and creative ways for RNs to achieve them and demonstrate that they have made a transition to the professional level of practice. Faculty must be knowledgeable and competent to make this kind of qualitative judgment. In addition, some course content does not easily lend itself to a decision about whether it has or has not been adequately covered in the previous program—for example, material relating to current issues and political and economic aspects of health care delivery.

## RNs Only

Second-step (sometimes erroneously called upper-division) programs for RNs imply that the first step has been either an associate degree or a diploma (Figure 7.3). Instructors are challenged to make content relevant to the RNs' experiences by acknowledging and utilizing what they bring to the program. Adult education principles can be applied to teaching methodology. Terminal objectives, although required to be consistent with those of the National League for Nursing for baccalaureate programs, can in fact be accomplished in more challenging ways and can be attained in greater depth with students who have actually practiced nursing before entering the program.

This type of program offers a ready-made peer support group sharing similar work, family, and back-to-school problems. However, this peer group can also be a powerful negative influence when all expectations are not met and resocialization is resisted (Woolley, 1978).

Many programs for RNs only are located in small liberal arts colleges that have no other health or professional programs. When college/university faculty and administrators have only a limited understanding of nursing in general and RN/BSN programs in particular, the program itself may suffer a lack of resources. In other situations, some see nurses as a ready-made market for declining student demand in certain liberal arts and humanities courses. The concept that nurses who are already licensed need to learn more nursing and have supervised practice at a level different from the one they have previously learned is difficult for some college/university administrators to grasp.

Another disadvantage of this educational model is that the programs are frequently offered in evening colleges or under the adult education administrative units. Although this may facilitate scheduling for adult learners and possibly offer some other advantages, unfortunately, it often means that program and student status within the college is not equal to that of the mainstream programs and may add another barrier to the resource allocation effort.

## Two Plus Two

Some schools have purposefully designed a two-step process; an associate degree is awarded after the first 2 years, and recipients sit for the licensing examination. They may then exit to the work world and/or continue on for the baccalaureate. This design clearly follows the model depicted in Figure 7.3; nursing content is differentiated into upper and lower divisions, and the terminal objectives of both programs are clear. Challenges are not usually necessary for students pursuing the baccalaureate, and no lower-division content need be repeated.

Although this is an organized and purposeful scheme, it presents other difficulties because the comprehensive baccalaureate approach cannot be taught from the beginning. Produced in the first 2 years is a technical nurse who must later be assisted in making a transition to a professional level of practice, thereby introducing an unnecessary hurdle to be overcome. The recent high school graduate who enters the lower division is immediately submerged in a heavy course load of basic science and nursing with accompanying laboratory requirements and has little opportunity to enjoy college activities and to assimilate the arts and humanities that are the hallmark of professional education.

Although students may enter these programs intending to complete all 4 years, many decide after becoming licensed that it is not necessary to do so, thereby adding to the supply of technical nurses rather than increasing the more acutely needed professional supply. However, transfer students who are graduates of diploma programs and other associate degree programs can sometimes be admitted to the upper division to replace those who choose not to go on.

## External Degrees

The external baccalaureate programs offered by the state universities of New York, New Jersey, and, in a modified form, by the California State Consortium, have grown in popularity, at least in part because of their convenience and cost-effectiveness. Nurses with associate degrees complete or test for a prescribed number of non-nursing credits and challenge all of the baccalaureate nursing content. Study guides for independent mastery of the material are supplied, but no personal instruction is provided. Clinical performance tests with clearly delineated critical behaviors must also be passed before the degree is awarded; these tests take several days and are conducted by carefully trained evaluators.

Supporters of this method of validation believe that knowledge and skills can be acquired in various ways other than formal study and that persons who possess these competencies should have the opportunity to demonstrate them by means of carefully constructed reliable tests. Convenience and cost-effectiveness for students, their employing agencies, and society are other advantages.

Objections to the external degree are based primarily on the lack of opportunity for socialization as well as the lack of consistent behavioral observation over an extended period of time, which is considered an integral part of college or university nursing education.

## RN/MSM

A fairly recent development has been a shortened path or track for the RN who wishes to earn both the baccalaureate and master's degrees. This RN/MSN program usually attempts to eliminate duplication of course work by using master's level courses to meet the requirements for the baccalaureate. Since many nursing master's degrees require more credits than others offered by the college or university, this is a logical and efficient arrangement. It is a cost-effective way for RNs to enter and remain in the system of higher education through the process of acquiring an undergraduate and a graduate degree.

However, NLN criterion 33 for the evaluation of baccalaureate and higher-degree programs in nursing, as revised in 1988, specifies that "The curriculum [for the master's degree] builds on the knowledge and competencies of baccalaureate education in nursing and provides for the attainment of advanced knowledge of nursing and related theories and their application to advanced nursing practice" (NLN, 1988). One of the purposes of this criterion is to assure that RNs studying for the master's degree do not bypass the baccalaureate and that there is adequate provision for effecting transition to the professional level of practice.

## Single-Purpose Institutions

An emerging issue in RN education is the function of single-purpose institutions, former diploma schools that have become regionally accredited to award the bachelor's degree. In order to meet NLN criteria for accreditation, these institutions are upgrading their faculty and changing their curricula to upper-division junior- and senior-year models. Students complete at least half of the degree requirements—usually the sciences, arts, and humanities—in a multipurpose institution before entering the nursing program as juniors. Because many former graduates of these institutions will be returning for the degree, the content of the new program will have to be clearly differentiated to avoid duplication and to provide for resocialization.

## COST-EFFECTIVENESS

The question of the best route to professional nursing is frequently considered in terms of comparative cost. A two-step process in which the RN can work after obtaining the associate degree in a low-cost community college, with the cost of the second step borne by the health care system, that is, the employing agency as a benefit, is more efficient for the individual than having the student bear the entire cost of the 4 years. However, others believe, that if nursing is to improve its professional standing and meet society's increasingly sophisticated nursing needs, the majority of its practitioners must be educated initially at this level. Society as a whole should bear the necessary cost through grants, scholarships, and loan-forgiveness programs.

Many nurse educators believe that all special RN educational programs should be discontinued to encourage a one-step unified model of professional education. They fear that perpetuating special programs for RNs, wherever they are placed and however they are designed, may encourage a two-step norm and remove nursing education from the mainstream of university life.

In summary, RN students have many choices to make when deciding on a nursing career and program. Practically speaking, the choices may be limited and dependent on cost and proximity of the educational institution. The program's educational philosophy may emerge much later, after the choice has been made, and may be the basis of dissatisfaction with the entire program.

RN educators also have a choice of how the programs they offer will be structured. A clear understanding of how the program's educational philosophy defines the relationship of technical and professional education will make curriculum decisions easier and avoid any confusion of purpose being transmitted to students.

## REFERENCES

Kelly, L. Y. (1985). *Dimensions of professional nursing* (5th ed.) New York: Macmillan.

National League for Nursing. (1982). *Position statement on educational mobility*. New York: Author.

National League for Nursing. (1988). *Criteria for the evaluation of baccalaureate and higher degree programs in nursing*. New York: Author.

Rapson, M. F. (1987). *Collaboration for articulation: RN to BSN*. New York: Author.

Rapson, M. F., Perry, L. A., and Parker, B. (1988, November). *Evaluation of selected academic outcomes of senior registered nursing students who have chosen three different advanced placement options available in the Maryland Nursing Articulation Model.* Poster presentation, Council of Baccalaureate and Higher Degree Programs, Cincinnati, Ohio.

Rogers, M. E. (1964). *Reveille in nursing.* Philadelphia: F. A. Davis.

Rogers, S. (1976). Testing the RN student's skills. *Nursing Outlook, 24*(7), 446–449.

Woolley, A. (1978). From RN to BSN: Faculty perceptions. *Nursing Outlook, 26*(2), 103–108.

Woolley, A. (1984). The bridge course: Transition to professional practice. *Nurse Educator, 9*(4), 15–19.

# 8

# Issues Surrounding RN/BSN Education: A View from Nursing Service

Maryann F. Fralic, R.N., M.N., Dr.P.H.

The "movement" of RNs returning to academe for the bachelor's degree is one that is welcome and observed with interest in nursing service settings. One cannot claim that this is a new phenomenon, because diploma and associate degree nurses have a long history of returning to school to earn the bachelor's degree. However, the numbers of nurses now pursuing this path have steadily increased. The reasons are multiple, ranging from esoteric to pragmatic; however, they are all applauded. The profession, the service settings, and most important, the patients who require nursing care will be well served by an expanded number of nurses with a broader educational base.

My perspective on this topic is that of a practicing nurse executive with responsibility for the patient care system in a complex and expanding academic health center. The views and opinions I express herein have been shaped and developed over time by observing large numbers of nurses in practice, listening to their professional concerns and difficulties, and engaging in frequent discussions with nurses as they deliberate their career and academic choices. Undoubtedly, my opinions have also been influenced by initially being a diploma nurse who returned for the BSN degree years ago. So this is not a new phenomenon; rather, it now has new dimensions and implications and merits examination. The question of educational alternatives for RNs has been and must continue to be a prime professional issue.

## ENVIRONMENTAL SCAN

Discussion of the RN/BSN phenomenon is difficult without first considering the context in which it occurs. The entire health care system has literally been reshaped in the past few years, and these changes will continue in the predictable future. This redesign presents nursing with the potential for increased opportunity and responsibility. Technology and knowledge are expanding exponentially, and the complexity of patient care requirements and the environment in which that care is delivered have dramatically increased.

With major growth in the elderly population, nursing needs can only increase. As some diseases are conquered, others emerge. The AIDS crisis is a classic example, presenting unprecedented requirements for expert, sensitive nursing care. The acute-care settings become ever more intense, and the intermediate and long-term-care settings are expanding and utilizing increasing numbers of nurses. Nontraditional patient care environments continue to develop. All of these factors portend complex, nurse-intensive systems.

The health care system can be accurately described as chaotic, evolving, market-driven, and responsive to the most cost-effective provider who can assure quality patient outcomes. Many feel that the professional nurse is well-positioned and prepared to be preeminent in this future system. However, just when it appears obvious that we will need an expanding and continuing stream of well-prepared nurses, we have a corresponding dilemma in the available manpower pool.

Like other professions, nursing has suffered a decline in the overall number of available traditional students. Additionally, nursing must aggressively compete for students with many other professions. As numbers of graduating nurses have declined, the demand for nursing services has escalated. As the demand for more sophisticated and better-prepared professional nurses increases, the need to prepare those nurses very well becomes more urgent.

## WHAT DOES IT MEAN?

The combined factors of escalating knowledge and complexity plus increasing demand mandate that we provide for sufficient numbers of appropriately prepared registered nurses to meet the nation's needs for nursing care. Our patients of today and tomorrow need and deserve nurses who have solidly based educational preparation, ample opportunity for educational advancement, and an expanded base of knowledge. An increasing number of well-prepared nurses is essential.

In discussing systems for advancement from RN/BSN, of first importance is to note that the majority of RNs have been and continue to be prepared at the associate degree level. As diploma education continues to decline, nursing has two predominant educational programs for preparing the beginning nurse: the bachelor's and associate degree programs. The large numbers of diploma nurses in practice have historically sought and will likely continue to seek access to baccalaureate programs. However, as diploma schools continue to close or merge with other programs, the number of diploma nurses will diminish steadily over time. Because the majority of nurses are prepared at the associate degree level, those students will, on a continuing basis, require access to solid, articulated, and receptive baccalaureate programs. Additionally, it may be viewed as a professional responsibility and in our collective best interest to smooth the way for those nurses who have diploma or associate degree training to achieve the bachelor's degree.

The BSN is sought by RNs for a wide variety of reasons. Frequently, the workplace has set the BSN as the standard or minimum requirement for advanced positions. In many hospitals, promotion to assistant head nurse, and certainly to head nurse, cannot occur without the bachelor's degree. This is no longer true just of academic health centers but is also a requirement in many community hospitals. Positions other than management positions in the workplace may also require the baccalaureate as minimum preparation. Thus, in addition to the profession itself citing the BSN as desired standard entry-level preparation, the workplace has also set its requirements.

The BSN graduate is often preferred by nursing service organizations for staff nurse positions. If one believes that education does indeed make a difference, then the BSN nurse should bring an additional knowledge base and an added level of professional performance. Indeed, in discussions with peers, nurse executives often will gauge the professionalism of one another's staff by the percentage of baccalaureate graduates as a proportion of overall RN staff.

What we have then is a health care system with expanding demand, an increasing number of RNs seeking the bachelor's degree, and an increasing number of service agencies seeking the baccalaureate graduate. And as most schools of nursing must now recruit aggressively to maintain sufficient numbers of students to preserve the vitality and strength of their programs, these schools have new opportunities to attract the RN student.

## THOUGHTS ABOUT SOME ETHICAL DIMENSIONS OF EDUCATION

It is important to acknowledge that there have been and continue to be value judgments and a negative bias by some against "technical education," that is, the education provided at the associate degree level. In my opinion, this has been internally destructive and divisive for nursing and is particularly perplexing because the majority of nurses are prepared at the technical level. I believe it becomes incumbent on the profession to provide every opportunity for these nurses should they desire to advance their education. Boyle (1972) related this very clearly in a statement of belief from the faculty of the College of Nursing at the University of Nebraska as follows: "Students who are beginning their education in any given discipline should have the right to progress within that discipline to the limits of their ability."

The bias against "technical nurses" is of long standing. Many years ago, a dean of a college of nursing was firm in her belief that "you cannot have a professional nurse unless they begin in a professional program. You cannot 'inject' the professionalism later on." This view, in my experience, is still held by others today and is an attitude that simply will not help nursing. Again, most nurses are prepared at a technical level; does that mean therefore that our profession will limit its own members in their desire to achieve professional status? The concept of terminal education is anathema to most thoughtful persons, and yet that is precisely what such an attitude implies. As long as we have fully sanctioned several pathways for entry into practice, I believe that we must provide clearly articulated and educationally sound programs between them.

Whether that articulation occurs as downward or upward meshing of curriculum, as described by Stevens (1981), is not the issue for this discussion; rather, it is how one conceptualizes the articulation between associate degree and BSN programs. The Venn diagrams that Stevens utilizes to depict the logical possibilities in the relationships between technical and professional programs are especially useful in conceptualizing this concept. One diagram depicts technical nursing as a part of professional nursing. This conceptualization enables one to acknowledge that nursing indeed does have techniques and technical skills that are integral to patient care. All nurses must possess these skills if patient care is to be safe and competent. Purists may say that professionalism is the substrata, and technical skills are thereafter incorporated. Pragmatists may see a nurse with high technical skills reentering the educational process to acquire the professional infrastructure. Happily, schools of nursing increasingly are preparing themselves to accept RN students who are eagerly seeking this professional infrastructure.

The nursing profession needs to acknowledge the academic legitimacy of all programs that are educationally sound and accredited. The profession's task is to link those programs in a manner that assures the achievement of appropriate educational outcomes as well as the academic growth and development of the individual learner. The RN student presents to academe as an adult learner with unique needs and contributions and with significant prior learning and experience. Responsive educational settings are increasingly developing programs to accommodate this particular student population. Lindsey (1988) summarizes this concept nicely in the following statement:

Each of us has a role in clarifying and strengthening the educational system for nursing and in implementing a rational coordinated system of establishing credentials for nursing. We need to consider a more systematic, deliberate approach for the diverse range of practice and the ever increasing number of specialties and subspecialties. (p. 72)

Clearly, more in-depth understanding of the scientific and theoretical basis for nursing practice will be essential in all future care settings, a need more urgent today than in 1974, when Kelly criticized a lack of commitment toward expediting career advancement in nursing education. She suggested that "if nursing ignored this clear-cut social movement, it may well be forced into less desirable patterns by the pressures of society" (Kelly, 1974). Thus, nursing has a history of seeking an expanded knowledge base of its members, and colleges of nursing today appear to be making even stronger efforts meet the needs of the members of our profession and ultimately the needs of society.

## UNIQUENESS OF THE RN STUDENT— SOME OBSERVATIONS

Nurse executives in the practice settings employ large numbers of nurses and have ample opportunity to interact with them, observe them, and listen to their concerns. The following comments are based on my own observations, over a period of years, of nurses who elect to become RN students in pursuit of the bachelor's degree. These observations, as they relate to group attributes, are substantiated by Campaniello (1988) in a recent study about professional nurses returning to school. These nurses are adult students, many of them are married, many are parents, and the vast majority of them are employed on either a full-time or part-time basis, frequently in very demanding and stressful jobs. They often make significant contributions by involvement in their communities. They are indeed multirole individuals. Many of them elected an associate degree or diploma program as initial nursing education because of its efficiency in time, access, or cost.

The fact that they elect to move from the certainty of the job situation and their competency in that situation to academe and its uncertainty reflects, I believe, a true seriousness of purpose. This appears to be amply demonstrated by their willingness to reenter academic life and accept significant incremental personal responsibilities.

Motivations for seeking the BSN are highly varied. For some it is strictly pragmatism: They want to qualify for the next promotion and are determined to meet the requirements. Some may simply be seeking self-development, personal growth, and enrichment. Others may have a serious commitment to the profession of nursing and a desire to remain in practice as a nurse over time, and they are seeking expanded knowledge and their next credential. Others experience a quiet peer pressure and seek to have their preparation perceived to be equal to their BSN colleagues. Others state, even before beginning their BSN program, that their goal is graduate education, and they see the baccalaureate as the interim degree. Whatever the motivation, we administrators attempt always to acknowledge and support that decision in the service setting. It is seldom an economic incentive for the nurse because salaries do not change in most settings when the nurse completes the program of study and remains in the same position. Those nurses are to be applauded for assuming significant academic commitment.

Campaniello's (1988) study treats the concept of role strain and the sources of conflict for nurses returning to school, noting that increased social supports for these students result in less perceived role conflict. We in the service settings, as well as those in the educational settings, need to be cognizant of the multiple strains and stresses that the RN student may experience. I know of no quiet undemanding practice arenas today. Cassells (Cassells, Redman, & Jackson, 1986) reports that approximately 90% of all baccalaureate students are employed; they are indeed a unique student population. Another obvious fact, but important to state, is that these students have already passed the RN licensing exam and have met requirements for practice. Most will have experience, ranging from minimal to extensive, as practicing nurses. Most will have internalized the nurse role. Some will bring with them other experiences, perhaps as managers of care. Others bring significant specific areas of advanced clinical prowess and expertise.

A relatively recent occurrence is that these prospective students now see themselves as bona fide customers and "shop around" extensively before selecting a BSN program, assuming that there are options and more than one school in their area. I have spoken with many nurses who seek information from a number of schools, and they visit and interview the schools to see which particular program will best accommodate them. I recently spoke with a highly skilled clinician who is a staff nurse with us from Australia. She interviewed at multiple schools and finally selected the one that she said "really wanted to help me get my degree." Hers is not an unusual story. Nurses returning for the BSN seem to be looking for the school that will welcome them as accomplished practicing nurses, not as novices. They are behaving as motivated, perceptive, and discriminating consumers. They are unwilling to tolerate programs that they believe consist of endless roadblocks. In discussing these problems with several of our staff nurses recently, I was reminded of a comment that a fellow student made some years ago while we were both trying to complete the doctoral program. He said, "I don't mind jumping through hoops, as long as there are holes in them."

I am pleased to note that there has been great effort on the part of schools of nursing in our state to attract and accommodate the RN student. One realistic dimension of this responsiveness, of course, is that competition for these students is sharpening as schools of nursing confront declining enrollment. However, there also seems to be an enthusiastic awareness that these nurses add a fine and unique dimension to the academic milieu.

## Observation of "Smart Moves" by Schools of Nursing

The following are some things that staff nurses have commented favorably on as they pursue the schools that will provide their baccalaureate education. This listing is not inclusive, nor is it ordered according to importance. It is merely a listing of the things that nurses have said that they liked about the schools they selected.

• The school acknowledged that the RN student was unique.

- The school marketed specifically to each segment of students (generic, RN, graduate) much like Proctor & Gamble, for example, marketed and prepared specific approaches, business plans, and programs for each of its product lines.
- The school actively marketed to the prospective RN student.
- RN students were treated as a rich resource.
- The school went to hospitals and other work sites to market their programs and recruit students.
- The school, in the student's view, developed an appropriate curriculum for them.
- The school went to hospitals and other work settings to conduct on-site classes.
- Classes were offered at convenient times for working nurses.
- The school had what the student perceived to be "good and fair" transfer/challenge policies.
- Personalized advisement was available for each student.
- A master study design and course plans were tailored for each student according to that student's needs.
- Specific attention was paid to socializing the student into the school, the overall curriculum, and the professional role.
- The RN student was treated with full legitimacy in the school and was viewed as a valuable asset to both generic students and to their own peer group.

I am reminded, as competition for these students increases, of a doctoral program designed for practicing nurse executives that may have some lessons for RN/BSN programs. The doctoral program is specifically designed with busy professionals in mind. Books are purchased for the students; articles are not placed on reserve but are reproduced and handed out at appropriate times; students are not required to wait in long lines to register, and so on. All of this may sound highly nontraditional and unrealistic; however, the program is clearly designed to market to and attract achieving professionals who have multiple commitments and demanding careers. Can we not take some of those lessons and apply them to the working RN student? RN students frequently have responsibilities to a spouse and/or children, a community, and very often a full-time or part-time position. Are there ways that schools can conserve student time and energy in order to maximize these students' educational experience and knowledge acquisition?

If faculty, school administration, and nursing service administration believe that these are valuable students to whom we all have an educational and professional responsibility, then we will do whatever is necessary to augment the educational process.

## Observation of "Smart Moves" by Nursing Service Organizations

Some of the strategies employed in nursing service settings appear to have been successful in encouraging and facilitating RNs' return for their bachelor's degree. Again, the list is not inclusive, nor is it ordered in any manner. Some of the successful strategies are as follows:

- The philosophy of the institution and its nursing division is one that values education and well-prepared professionals and actively supports those efforts and activities.
- Tuition assistance and scholarship programs are available for employees.
- Flexible and accommodating scheduling facilitates course work.
- Psychological support and encouragement are provided for the nurse throughout the process.
- The RN's academic experience is augmented or enhanced in whatever manner possible.
- Educational leaves or sabbaticals are offered to facilitate academic program completion.
- Opportunities to apply school content to active practice are sought so that the student's efforts are reaffirmed during the educational process.
- Students' achievement and academic success is acknowledged.

It has been particularly important to encourage nurse managers to support the RN student in every possible way. Sometimes this is highly inconvenient—days off may change, patient care coverage can become more complicated, some may have to change their work shift for a particular period, and so on. A different scenario occurs when nurse managers themselves are the RN students. The scope of their job responsibilities, plus multiple demands on their time, may preclude flexible scheduling to meet class schedules. Extra sensitivity and responsiveness to the needs of this group are warranted.

At our hospital, we believe that the better prepared each of us is, the better the entire nursing division becomes. So we must fully support the working student. We then celebrate their achievements through recognition ceremonies, articles published in hospital newsletters, and many other ways of recognition and reinforcement that are so essential. We believe that their individual achievement is also our collective achievement.

## Some "Not So Smart" Moves by Nursing Service Organizations

With few exceptions, nursing service settings have not differentiated practice between the professional and technical level of nurse. There has been no differentiation in roles or in responsibilities. There is no distinction in the work between nurses prepared in the various levels of education. This absence of delineation has hampered the process of clarity of practice within the profession. One might argue about whether it is the responsibility of the educational process or the practice environment to activate and operationalize this distinction. However, it is obviously a shared responsibility that has not been met, and that must be addressed in the near future. Because no distinction has been made between the work of the two levels of nurse, very little distinction in salary exists. A system for differentiation would clearly address both the work and the remuneration issues.

## THE BENEFITS OF RN/BSN EDUCATION FOR THE SERVICE SETTING

It is in nursing's collective interest to encourage advanced education for nurses at all levels. Intellectually stimulated staff members are a wonderful and challenging resource! In a recent survey of staff nurses that we conducted at our institution, the satisfier that our RN staff listed as number one was "the competence of peers" (Robert Wood Johnson University Hospital, 1988). That to us was indeed a powerful statement that surpassed salary, scheduling, benefits, and all of the other typical answers that one might expect. What it says is that professionals want and value good colleagues and that the presence of competent and well-prepared colleagues is a major satisfier.

and acquire a conceptual base for professional practice, they apply the nursing process more comprehensively, and there is a more consistent application of a theoretical basis for practice. Patients need and will increasingly require more knowledgeable nurses planning and delivering their care. The needs of clinical practice mandate that we facilitate advanced education in every way possible. Thus, there are multiple important driving forces for facilitating RN/BSN programs. The marketplace, the profession, and patient care needs are all potent stimuli. Our collective professional responsibility is to smooth the way.

## SPECULATING ON THE FUTURE

Coincidentally, another impetus for increasing articulation among nursing programs comes from recurring nursing shortages. Many strategies are being formulated and forwarded by various organizations, commissions, and groups to increase nursing manpower. A strong repeated recommendation is that nursing must attract increasing numbers of both traditional and nontraditional students. Second-career students, persons already employed in health care positions (such as nursing assistants, licensed practical nurses, EMTs, etc.) and older adult students are cited as potential nursing candidates. Casting this wider net for students will increasingly require that schools prepare for articulated programs in a manner that facilitates the entry and progression of every qualified candidate.

This change, combined with a health care environment that demands increasing levels of nursing knowledge, workplaces that set the BSN as the necessary credential for many positions, and a steady stream of associate degree graduates, mandate that solid AD/ BSN programs develop. Technically prepared nurses will increasingly matriculate into professional nursing programs. Perhaps we will see more of the concept of meshing curriculum that Stevens (1981) describes as baccalaureate schools prepare themselves to accept more associate degree nurses and as associate degree programs seek to better prepare their graduates for progression into baccalaureate education.

Nursing now and in the future will need all of its academic programs to be educationally sound, with very high standards and expectations for all learners. Programs will become more "user friendly" as the nurse continues to be an increasingly discriminating and demanding consumer of academic services.

Nursing service organizations will be required to accommodate even larger numbers of working RN students, which will add to the complexity of scheduling and staffing these very intense and high-stress environments. The quid pro quo for the service organization is that the nursing staff becomes more scientifically based and thoughtful in its practice and that there is an increased professionalization of the entire nursing division.

Any discussion or debate of the factors surrounding RN/BSN education is indeed complex and sometimes contentious. However, my firm belief is that the profession of nursing will be strengthened and well served by our thoughtful, concerted, and reasoned approach to this very significant issue.

## REFERENCES

Boyle, R. E. (1972). Articulation: From associate degree through masters. *Nursing Outlook*, *20*(10), 670–672.

Campaniello, J. A. (1988). When professional nurses return to school: A study of role conflict and well-being in multiple-role women. *Journal of Professional Nursing*, *4*(2), 136–140.

Cassells, J. M., Redman, B. K., & Jackson, S. J. (1986). Generic baccaulaureate nursing student satisfaction regarding professional and personal development prior to graduation and one-year postgraduation. *Journal of Professional Nursing, 2*(2), 114–129.

Kelly, L. Y. (1974). Open curriculum, what and why. *American Journal of Nursing, 74*(12), 2238.

Lindsey, A. M. (1988). Strengths and challenges: Nursing in the 21st century [Editorial]. *Journal of Professional Nursing, 4*(2), 71–72.

Robert Wood Johnson University Hospital. (1988). *Registered nurse survey.* Unpublished.

Stevens, B. J. (1981). Program articulation: What it is and what it is not. *Nursing Outlook, 29*(12), 700–706.

# 9

# Development and Implementation of an RN-to-BSN Option at a Public Institution

Dorothy L. Powell, Ed.D., R.N.

This chapter discusses the development of an RN completion program at Norfolk State University in Norfolk, Virginia, a predominantly black institution. The incentives for starting this program were perhaps different from others discussed in this book because the program was inspired by the Virginia Plan to desegregate institutions of higher education in the state. Political issues and equal-access issues compounded the process of program development and implementation. These issues are discussed in the following section. The impact of the issues on the establishment of admission requirements, curriculum, learning experiences, scheduling, recruitment, faculty, and students are all discussed in succeeding portions of this chapter.

## BACKGROUND

During the late 1970s and early 1980s, a significant growth occurred in nursing education programs in institutions of higher education.

According to data from the National League for Nursing (NLN, 1988), between 1981 and 1986, 72 new bachelor's degree and 61 new associate degree programs started, accounting for a 15.8% and a 7% increase, respectively. These figures represent a 2.3% growth rate in bachelor's degree programs over the rate of growth between 1975 and 1980. By contrast, associate degree programs grew at a slower rate between 1981 and 1986 (7%) than between 1975 and 1980 (12.7%). Many of the new bachelor's degree programs initiated were specially designed for RNs. The NLN reports 159 such programs in 1986, compared with 452 generic baccalaureate programs.

The rise in the number of new programs during this period is related to several factors. One, of course, was the continuing requirement to upgrade nurses without bachelor's degrees. Less often recognized as a factor was the overall decline in enrollment in institutions of higher education. In the final report of the Carnegie Council on Policy Studies in Higher Education (1980), it was forecast that by 1997 institutions of higher education would experience a 23.3% decline in the number of 18–24-year-olds enrolling as undergraduates. Further, the report predicted that the enrollment decline would be offset in part by students over 25, thus yielding an overall decline of 19%.

Institutions of higher education embarked on many strategies to counter the anticipated decline. Among other things, it became fashionable to start nursing programs because nursing during this period was a very attractive discipline, generally bringing in more students than there were spaces in the classes. Also, advocacy by the nursing profession for the baccalaureate in nursing to be the entry requirement for professional practice inspired many institutions to start RN completion programs.

The creation of nursing programs was also viewed by some states as a partial solution to demands by the federal government to more fully integrate institutions of higher education. States such as Virginia and Louisiana were under court order at the turn of the decade to increase black enrollment in predominantly white institutions and to increase white enrollment at predominantly black institutions. Such was the fundamental inspiration for the creation of the baccalaureate program in nursing at Norfolk State University, a state-supported institution of higher education in Virginia that offered associate, bachelor's, and master's degrees.

The development of the program was layered with heavy political overtones. The baccalaureate program was conceived as an upper-level RN completion program that was to articulate with associate degree programs in neighboring, largely white community colleges. Ironically, Norfolk State also had an accredited associate degree program that was about 75% black and had a record of high success rates on the professional nursing licensing examination.

The associate degree program was the first of its type in Virginia and one of the original seven associate degree programs in the United States. The state's desegregation plan, formulated by the state coordinating body [The State Council of Higher Education of Virginia (SCHEV)], had a profound effect on how the associate degree program and its future were perceived as the state desegregation efforts gathered impetus. The associate degree program was supposed to be replaced by the conceived baccalaureate program. The rationale behind the strategy was that black students who would attend Norfolk State for the associate degree in nursing would turn to the largely white community college programs, thus increasing black enrollment in the community colleges. Likewise, the design of the RN program at Norfolk State would be attractive to white students by allowing graduates of the specific associate degree programs to articulate directly into the junior year of the baccalaureate program at Norfolk State.

The desire of SCHEV for Norfolk State to phase out its associate degree program in exchange for the baccalaureate program was not viewed favorably by the administration of Norfolk State. The historical significance of the program, along with its success in attracting and graduating students, was an important asset for the university and not something the university wished to give up for a new program of unknown capability. Thus, an alternate plan that allowed Norfolk State to retain its associate degree program in addition to beginning the BSN program was sought by the university. The negotiations to achieve agreement on such an alternative plan were a long and arduous process involving a variety of politically inspired maneuvers and appeal procedures.

Initially, the proposal to SCHEV for approval to establish the BSN program was delayed because the plan did not call for phasing out the associate degree program. Subsequent efforts by the university to retain the associate degree program were rejected despite extensive documentation that supported continuation of the program. One strategy advanced to respond to the continuing need for associate degree nursing education at Norfolk State was for one of the local community colleges to assume responsibility for associate degree education at Norfolk State, including teaching the required courses at Norfolk State. This proposal was short-lived. When it became evident that Norfolk State was adamant in its desire to start a BSN program, other area universities and colleges were brought into the debates. These schools were invited to comment on whether they believed the Tidewater area needed another BSN program (two other BSN programs existed at the time) such as that being proposed at Norfolk State and on the capability of community colleges to absorb more associate degree students into existing programs. Despite the continuous proliferation of counterstrategies, Norfolk State persisted in its efforts to gain approval.

Resolution of the positions of SCHEV and Norfolk State required ongoing negotiation and a considerable investment of time and effort on the part of state and university officials. The head of the nursing program was deeply involved in planning and strategy sessions at the university and in state-level meetings. Tremendous collaboration was required between the head of the nursing unit and the university administration. It became the responsibility of the nursing head to help the president and vice-president—who were the chief spokespersons and negotiators for the university in negotiations with the state coordinating body, the state legislature, and the U.S. Office of Civil Rights—to understand all of the nuances of baccalaureate education, the differences between baccalaureate education in nursing and associate degree and diploma nursing education, accreditation requirements, the myriad of professional issues confronting nursing, and various trends affecting health care, as well as local issues impacting on new nursing programs. Throughout the negotiations with state agencies to win the new program, a lot of learning occurred among the university's administration. This learning ultimately led to enhanced understanding of the needs of nursing education and its uniqueness, as well as the acquisition of solid support for the program.

An agreement was reached late in 1981, after nearly 2 years of negotiation, when the university won an appeal before the State

Council of Higher Education. The university was allowed to begin the RN program in January 1982 and continue the operation of the associate degree program. Funding sufficient to start the new programs was provided through a special appropriation from the state. The agreement also included a commitment to review both programs at a future date, when a decision would be made about the continuation of one or both programs.

## PROGRAM DEVELOPMENT

Among the factors that caused Norfolk State to persist in its efforts to win approval were those related to differences between associate degree students and RNs in a baccalaureate completion program.

The university's desire to retain the associate degree program was based, in part, on several principles that hold wisdom for anyone contemplating initiation of an RN completion program. First, students in an RN completion program are more likely to attend part-time than are associate degree students, who are more likely to attend full-time. Second, interested RNs differ in their academic readiness to begin the major in nursing; many will spend some time completing prerequisites before actually taking nursing courses. Third, the actual number of active students, the number of courses, and the number of required sections may be initially less in a new program than those needed in an active and successful continuing program. These principles, particularly the third—the concept of starting small and building on an as-need basis—posed difficulties for the university when it was asked to give up an established program for a new program. What would happen to the more than 300 new students at the university yearly seeking admission to the associate degree program? The financial and legal implications of a simple swap of programs did not justify agreement by the university to the original plan of deleting the associate degree program in exchange for the BSN program.

Simultaneous with long hours of high-level university efforts to win approval, the development of a quality program was an ongoing process. Based on the stated expectation of the articulation plan, an innovative program was developed that allowed for direct articulation with existing associate degree programs in three sites. Two of the associate degree programs, Tidewater Community College and Thomas Nelson Community College, were part of the state's community college system. The third was Norfolk State's own program. The articulation plan had to allow for academic hours earned in the associate degree program to be credited toward the baccalaureate. The plan also had to facilitate entry into the junior year, thereby producing what is commonly referred to as a 2 + 2 program. Built into the 2 + 2 program was development of a defensible system that did not require examination of previous nursing learning.

This last point, the concept that a registered practicing nurse should not have to undergo testing of her professional knowledge and skills, raised considerable questions and advice from nursing colleagues across the state and nationally. They believed that some form of individual validation of previous nursing knowledge had to be done. On the other hand, the arrangement needed to comply with the articulation model being proposed for other programs that were also part of the university's desegregation plan. In agreements between Norfolk State and Tidewater Community College, students completing associate degree programs had to be able to enter Norfolk State at the junior year without challenge exams. The generic articulation model did not require validation beyond evidence that certain courses in the community college had been completed successfully. The political pressures of the developmental process and this aspect in particular forced the nursing faculty to respond to the similarities nursing shares with other academic disciplines rather than advocating for its uniqueness, which has often occurred in nursing education when considering transfer credits.

## DEVELOPING ADMISSION REQUIREMENTS

One of the early activities of the faculty was to determine the basis of articulation and hence the requirements for admission to the baccalaureate program. The associate degree program at Norfolk State was to be the model or standard against which the other two programs would be evaluated. The Norfolk program had recently been accredited by the National League for Nursing and was known to produce high-level graduates with high first-time success on the licensing exam. The nursing faculties of each school met to compare and contrast their programs. During these in-depth meetings, philosophies, terminal objectives, conceptual frameworks, course objectives, learning experiences, and evaluation procedures and requirements were reviewed and documented. Based on this extensive review, a common core of knowledge, skills, and competencies held by graduates of the three programs was determined. In addition, it was noted that the required competencies were consistent with those listed in the *Competencies of Associate Degree Graduates* (NLN Publication No. 23-1731, 1978).

The review revealed that the community colleges and the associate degree program at Norfolk State had similar general education requirements. Graduates from all three programs had the equivalent of 6 semester hours of English; a minimum of 3 hours each of sociology, general psychology, and developmental psychology; 6–8 hours of anatomy and physiology; and varied numbers of electives. Norfolk State, the template school, had 4 credits of microbiology, whereas the two community colleges only required 2 credits. Only Norfolk State required physical education in its curriculum. Similar nursing credits were apparent among all programs with a range of 34–36 semester hours.

Minimum requirements that would constitute the admission standards and be transferable toward the BSN (see Table 9.1) were mutually agreed on by the three institutions. In addition, 34–36 credits of lower-level nursing were transferable.

Each school chose the date that their curriculum would be put into place. Only those students who graduated on or after that date would be allowed to receive transferable credits in nursing. Other students, as well as the anticipated number of registered nurses from nonarticulated schools, were required to take the five-part ACT-PEP examination (this was later changed to a three-part series: Differences in Nursing Care). Students who graduated from an articulated program had 5 years from the date of their graduation to begin coursework in the baccalaureate program or take the ACT-PEP series.

The currency of science credits was another decision dealt with under the articulation agreement. A limit of 10 years was set on all

## TABLE 9.1. Minimum Course Requirement for Admission

| Course | Credits |
|---|---|
| General psychology | 3 |
| Human development | 3 |
| Introductory sociology | 3 |
| Anatomy and physiology | 6 |
| Microbiology | 3[a] |
| English composition | 6 |
| U.S. history | 3 |
| Free elective | 3 |

[a]One community college changed its microbiology requirement to two 3-credit quarters, or the equivalent of 4 semester hours. Graduates of the other community college were required to take a microbiology course (3–4 semester hours) or a challenge exam.

college-credit science courses. For students who did not meet the age requirement, a 5-credit science update course was developed by the biology department. The course allowed students to become current in their knowledge of anatomy, physiology, and microbiology and included a lab. Students who had old college credits received credit on their transcripts once they successfully completed the update course. Students without previous college credits in the sciences (i.e., early diploma graduates) could use the science update course as a means of review prior to taking challenge exams provided by the biology department.

Students admitted to the program received 34–36 lower-division nursing credits by transfer or examination and 29 credits in science and general education courses. Thus, students entered the junior year with a minimum of 63 credits towards the BSN.

## DEVELOPING AND IMPLEMENTING THE CURRICULUM

The design of the curriculum was based on several beliefs the faculty held about associate degree and baccalaureate education.

1. Bachelor's and associate degree education in nursing are contingent on their relationship with a broad general education core. The curriculum should share in approximately equal parts coursework in nursing and general education.
2. Associate degree education in nursing has its emphasis in secondary care; baccalaureate education in nursing contains components of primary, secondary, and tertiary levels of nursing.
3. Baccalaureate education in nursing has a strong theory base and constitutes the basis of the nursing process.
4. Associate degree education in nursing operationalizes nursing and relates it to a theoretical foundation.
5. An understanding of the research process and utilization of research findings is an essential component of baccalaureate education but is not usually present in associate degree education.
6. Baacalaureate education prepares for beginning leadership and management in nursing within organized settings.

Given these basic assumptions reflecting differences between associate and baccalaureate education, it was the faculty's belief that an upper-level baccalaureate program could be developed that stressed primary and tertiary care while enhancing secondary care.

The organization and sequencing of the baccalaureate curriculum were developed from the philosophy, purposes, and objectives of the program. The upper-level curriculum was organized into a possible four-semester course of study. However, because the typical student was envisioned to be employed full-time as a registered nurse, the curriculum design allowed study on a part-time basis, although total matriculation time was not to exceed 5 years from the first nursing course to receipt of the degree.

Despite adopting a flexible schedule, a required sequence of courses was determined (Table 9.2).

The upper-level curriculum consisted of 30 general education credits and 35 nursing credits for a total of 65 credits. Thus, with the 63 transfer credits, the baccalaureate called for a minimum of 128 credits.

The faculty believed that a successful career mobility program

**TABLE 9.2. Required Sequence of Courses**

| Course | Credits |
| --- | --- |
| Junior year | |
|   Chemistry | 8 |
|   Statistics | 3 |
|   Principles of speech or advanced communication skills | 3 |
|   Business management | 3 |
|   Literature of the Western world | 3 |
|   Socialization seminar | 1 |
|   Health assessment | 3 |
|   Concepts and theories of nursing | 2 |
|   Multiculturalism/bioethics | 2 |
|   Principles of community health nursing | 2 |
|   Community health nursing | 4 |
| Senior year | |
|   Pathophysiology | 3 |
|   Music or art appreciation | 3 |
|   U.S. history or Western civilization | 3 |
|   Group process in nursing | 2 |
|   Advanced clinical nursing (child rearing/childbearing) | 5 |
|   Advanced clinical nursing (crisis/crisis intervention) | 5 |
|   Nursing research | 2 |
|   Nursing leadership/management | 3 |
|   Senior seminar | 1 |
|   Nursing elective | 2 |
|   Free elective | 3 |

for RNs included more than an articulated curriculum. Of equal importance were matters pertaining to format and accessibility of courses. Hence, an early commitment was made by the faculty to offer courses at times and in structures compatible with the work schedules of the anticipated student pool.

Thus, a variety of patterns were used, many based on suggestions from students. The entire curriculum, with the exception of some nursing clinical experiences, was available after 4 P.M. and/or on weekends. The cooperation of other areas of the university made such scheduling possible. Nursing and non-nursing courses were offered on single evenings, as opposed to the traditional format of offering courses on two or three evenings per week. As an example, a chemistry lecture could be taken on Monday, statistics on Tuesday, two or three nursing courses on Thursday, and other general education courses on remaining evenings.

Clinical experiences that averaged 9 hours per week were either offered 1 day a week and/or concentrated into 2 days (or evenings) per week for half a semester. For instance, the senior course in crisis and crisis intervention utilized 1 day and 1 evening experience of 8 hours each, covering half of the semester. The management experience was concentrated into 6 8-hour days covering 2 weeks. Students typically use vacation time for this experience. In addition, some clinical experiences were scheduled on weekends.

Other nontraditional approaches to didactic courses included workshop formats. Some 2-hour courses met on weekends, using large blocks of time and multiple teaching strategies. For example, one section of a nursing theory course met for 6 hours on four Saturdays spaced throughout the semester. Another senior seminar course concentrated its time into a 2-week format near the end of the semester.

## CLINICAL EXPERIENCES

The philosophy of the program and its conceptualization speaks to a program that fosters application of the nursing process to clients in a variety of settings. The emphasis of the program is on primary and tertiary care with an enhancement of secondary care. These are the philosophical underpinnings of the program, and course design and related clinical experiences were determined with these philosophical beliefs in mind. For instance, students enrolled in community health nursing had experiences in industrial settings, penal institutions, home health agencies, and other community settings in addition to traditional health department experiences. Students in advanced clinical nursing (child rearing/childbearing) cared for pregnant clients in migrant labor camps on the Eastern Shore of Virginia, pregnant teens in low-income public housing projects, and chronic and terminally ill children in a hospice. Students in crisis/crisis intervention spent three consecutive evenings in the emergency room, conducted health assessments and teaching sessions with homeless individuals in temporary shelters, worked with recently discharged mental patients in halfway houses, and made calls with the city's rescue unit.

Students were involved in selecting some learning experiences to meet their individual goals and interests. For instance, one student who worked as a supervisor in a general hospital wanted to enhance her knowledge and skills in pediatric nursing. A 3-week (40 hours/week) instructional/preceptorial experience was planned for her at a tertiary pediatric hospital. Another student planned and taught a course of several weeks' duration on hypertension to groups of women in inner-city churches; she successfully reached her goal when the churches adopted an ongoing blood pressure watch/advisement program.

The program adhered to adult learning principles and involved students thoroughly in ongoing planning and evaluation. The roles of teacher and learner were more shared in this approach than is often evident in generic programs. However, despite the level of independence students had in their own learning, all clinical experiences were guided by faculty to assist students in achieving the high level of clinical competence, problem solving, and critical thinking expected.

## THE FACULTY

The initial faculty for the baccalaureate program were drawn from long-standing associate degree faculty. The department head had a master's degree in maternal–child nursing and was completing a doctorate in administration of higher education. A second faculty member held a master's degree in medical-surgical nursing and was also completing her doctorate in administration of higher education. The third member of the team was prepared at the master's level in community mental health nursing. She too was engaged in doctoral study. The final initial faculty member held a master's degree in community health nursing.

This group of faculty initially took on the responsibility of curriculum development while carrying full-time teaching loads in the associate degree program. Every Monday for more than a year, the group met off-campus at one member's home to work on the curriculum from 9 A.M. until 4 P.M. It was necessary to get away from the work environment to be able to concentrate exclusively on the creative work to be done. The group worked well together, and the curriculum became truly a unification of the ideas of the group.

By the beginning of the second year, the curriculum had been completed, approved by the University Curriculum Committee, and clinical placements secured. However, consensus had not been reached with the state coordinating body over the terms of the agreement. Thus, the university was prevented from starting the program in the fall of 1981. In November 1981, a successful appeal was made before the SCHEV. The program was granted permission to begin in the spring of 1982, and the associate degree program was allowed to continue.

Once approval had been achieved, additional faculty were hired. Initially, two faculty members were hired in the associate degree program to grant 50% release time to the original group of faculty, who would now be sharing their teaching time between the two programs. In addition, a full-time counselor-recruiter was hired. Within another 6 months, a maternal–child health faculty member was hired to become responsible for the child rearing/childbearing course in the second-year curriculum and for leadership-management. This faculty member was prepared at the master's level in maternal–infant nursing and had extensive experience as a clinical nurse specialist and administrator in two major pediatric hospitals. The community mental health faculty member was appointed coordinator of the baccalaureate program.

## THE STUDENTS AND RECRUITMENT

The initial class of four students entered in January 1982 following approval of the program by SCHEV the previous November. All were white and consisted of three females and one male RN. Three were recent graduates of the associate degree program at Norfolk State, and one was an associate degree graduate of Thomas Nelson Community College. All attended full-time and wanted to complete the program by spring 1983. Therefore, the second semester curriculum was taught during the summer of 1982, allowing three of the four to graduate in June 1983.

The controversy surrounding approval of the program and the uncertainty as to when it would begin contributed to the small size of the initial class. However, interest remained high. Approximately 20 to 30 students were identified who were meeting requirements for admission or taking general education courses in the baccalaureate curriculum to lighten their load once admitted. By fall 1982, eight new students were admitted, four blacks and four whites. One student was a diploma graduate and successfully completed the ACT-PEPs on first testing. The others were associate degree graduates from the articulated schools.

To enhance enrollment, the health assessment course was offered to any RN regardless of admission status. This was used as an incentive and recruitment tactic. The course was offered at several off-campus sites in surrounding rural and urban communities. RNs not admitted to the program were assured that the course would count toward the BSN at Norfolk State as long as they were admitted within 5 years of the date the course was taken. During the initial application of this strategy, three sections were offered. By the following fall, 21 new students entered the program (third entering class) maintaining about a 50-50 black-white racial composition.

Hospitals in the region were targeted as primary recruitment sites. The counselor/recruiter visited these agencies regularly and evaluated nurses' prior education on site. Applications for admission were also accepted during these visits.

A unique relationship developed with one rural hospital, Louise Obici Hospital in Suffolk, Virginia. This hospital, located some 30 miles from Norfolk, had a long-standing diploma program. The hospital administrator and nursing school director expressed a desire to have their graduates continue their education into a baccalaureate program. They were interested in working with Norfolk State to facilitate easy access and credit for previous learning. An agreement was reached between the two institutions to work toward a unique articulation arrangement. The director of the diploma program and the chairman of the Norfolk State program were assigned the responsibility of working out the details of the arrangement.

A series of meetings was held, and the following items were agreed to; they differed somewhat from the elements of the agreement with the community colleges.

1. Several changes were made in the general education and science requirements of the diploma program to bring them into line with the prerequisites of the RN/BSN program at Norfolk State. The diploma program used the resource of Paul D. Camp Community College, located in Suffolk, for all of its support courses. The additional courses specified under the agreement were available at the community college.

2. Students in the diploma program would take the three-part ACT-PEP exams (Differences in Nursing Care) during their last semester of study.

All other aspects of the agreement were similar to those specified in the agreement with the associate degree programs in the community colleges. This articulation arrangement was monumental and significant because it represented the first of its kind in Virginia between a public, predominately black university and a private, predominately white hospital. It also was unique in uniting a baccalaureate and a diploma program. The agreement was signed by the hospital administrator and the president of the university in the spring of 1987.

The formal network among articulated institutions constituted the most profitable recruitment mechanism and accounts for most of the students currently enrolled. However, the reputation of the graduates, the quality and diversity of learning experiences for students, and the accessibility of the program attracted many other students from throughout the region. The current enrollment is approximately 67, and the largest number of graduates, 21, completed the program in May 1988.

## SUMMARY

This chapter has addressed the development and implementation of an RN completion program in a public, predominantly black institution of higher education that articulates with associate degree programs in two predominantly white community colleges. The program was part of the desegregation plan for institutions of higher education in the Commonwealth of Virginia. The major controversy surrounding approval of the baccalaureate program by the state coordinating body centered on the stated position that the university should phase out its historically significant and successful associate degree program as part of the approval of the baccalaureate program. The position of the university was to retain the associate degree program and start the BSN program. After 2 years of negotiations and appeals, the coordinating body gave approval for the university to start the BSN program in 1982 and to retain its associate degree program, at least on a temporary basis, until another evaluation could be made several years later.

Now, 7 years later, Norfolk State University continues to operate both programs. Both are NLN- accredited and maintain strong enrollment patterns. The associate degree program has experienced no decline in enrollment and the BSN program has demonstrated steady growth. The student population is culturally diverse. The BSN program, in particular, attracts an equal proportion of black and white students.

Educationally, the articulation model is effective as a means of career mobility for RNs. The close working relationship between the university and the community colleges contributes to program quality and maintenance of a clear perspective on differences between associate degree and baccalaureate education. The natural feeder system for the baccalaureate program from the three associate degree programs ensures a rich applicant pool and maintenance of enrollment. Also, the program design allows for flexibility in course scheduling and formating as well as the opportunity for innovative teaching/learning strategies using a myriad of clinical experiences. The program is strong, effective, and very attractive. The successes experienced were well worth the efforts required to make it a reality. The program is a source of pride for the university, the community, and perhaps even the state of Virginia.

## REFERENCES

Carnegie Council and and Policy Studies in Higher Education. (1980). *Three thousand futures, the next twenty years for higher education* (final report, p. 37). San Francisco: Jossey-Bass.

National League for Nursing, Division of Research. (1988). *State approved schools of nursing RN 1988*, p. 5. New York: Author.

National League for Nursing. (1978). Competencies of associate degree graduates (Report No. 23-1731). New York: Author.

# 10

# Development and Implementation of an RN-to-BSN Option at a Private Institution

## Judith Ann Balcerski, Ph.D., R.N.

Immediate need rather than planned choice was the initial impetus for the development of the RN option at Barry University in 1978. Within the 12 months prior to the admission of the first students, two local universities had closed their doors to nurses. One, a state university, had been in existence for a number of years and had a large enrollment of several hundred students; when it closed the RN program, it left students stranded and disillusioned. The other, a private university, admitted RN students in September 1977 and closed the program 3 months later, also leaving a class in midstream. The dean of the latter program came to Barry University School of Nursing for help for her students.

At that time, the Barry University School of Nursing, founded in 1953, had about 200 students in a generic program (Basic Option) with classes of about 40 to 50 from freshman to senior years. This program was based on a fairly traditional medical model curriculum and had only rarely received RN applications because RNs' specific needs had been met by nearby institutions. Of the 14 full-time faculty members, all but one were prepared at the master's level in pertinent nursing specialties, were skilled practitioners, and enjoyed teaching traditional students in an institution that expected and rewarded excellence in teaching.

## NEED ASSESSMENT

A needs assessment was neither necessary nor timely in our situation. Although a university 20 miles south and one 30 miles north of Barry enrolled nurses, there was significant pressure on Barry from the local RN community to initiate a program. The closure of the two other university programs created a large number of interested and willing potential students. Not surprisingly, these students were somewhat suspicious of any program initiated ostensibly on their behalf. The stability of our program was crucial to recapture the goodwill and motivation of the RNs in the greater Miami area. We knew that, once implemented, the continuation of a program that met these students' needs, was NLN-accredited, and maintained educational integrity, was essential. Our immediate task was to assess our capabilities and the willingness of the faculty to undertake the option. We did not undertake implementation lightly but did move swiftly, admitting the first students in about 2 months.

The RN option implemented ten years ago barely resembles the RN option of today. The changes made during the intervening years were essential to maintain the currency of the program and to incorporate the principles of adult learning. The faculty and administrator of the School of Nursing originally developed this option by stepping off only slightly from what they understood and felt capable of doing. Gradually, as the faculty developed new skills and understood more clearly the needs of their students, they made changes in the option. Central to program changes was the concern of faculty for students, demonstrated by their ability to listen to the students and to move to meet their needs. The program of today presents a better model for implementation than that initiated 10 years ago, but the process of incremental change is an equally important factor in program planning. This chapter will describe the original and the current RN option from the perspective of a private university.

## RESOURCES

Prior to the implementation of the RN option in the School of Nursing, many nurses were turning to Barry's Division of Adult and Continuing Education (ACE) to earn the bachelor of professional studies (BPS) degree. This program was initiated to meet the needs of the working adult. Students developed a portfolio of noncredit nursing coursework and experience and were granted credits to a maximum of 60. With the addition of the remaining liberal arts courses, they were able to earn the BPS in a short and relatively painless way. Although this degree was appropriate for some nurses, many graduates soon began to realize that the BPS alone without the upper-level nursing competencies did not prepare them for direct access to many MSN programs, including that later developed at Barry.

Establishment of a new program at Barry in 1978 was based on the ability of the program to pay for at least its direct costs. Because the small number of new students in the RN option enrolled in the same courses as the basic-option students, the cost was anticipated to be minimal. These costs included salary for a part-time adviser and, later, additional clinical faculty. No further resources were originally required for library, audiovisual, or secretarial staff needs. Additional space was unnecessary because the part-time adviser was already employed in a faculty capacity. Recruitment for students was also unnecessary at this time.

During the 10 years of the program's existence (Fall 1978 to Spring 1989), enrollment has increased from 9 to 138 RNs taking prerequisite and nursing courses. One full-time director and a half-time adviser are now employed. About 2½ full-time-equivalent (FTE) faculty are teaching nurses in a separate track. Additional secretarial staff and administrative office space have been added as needed.

Then and now, advising RNs is the most important responsibility of the school to the students. At Barry, qualified students are admitted directly to the program of their choice. This means that both basic- and RN-option students begin being advised through the School of Nursing even as they take liberal arts courses. In fact, the adviser spends many hours assisting students who are inquiring about the program and students who intend to take their nursing courses at Barry but who are earning the prerequisites through College Level Examination Program (CLEP), proficiency tests, and correspondence courses, at Barry off-campus sites, or at another institution. Employing an adviser who has a keen interest in facilitating the success of adults and who has an acute understanding of academic requirements and the methods to fulfill them is imperative. A skillful and motivated adviser can encourage the nurse to overcome the two most important barriers to earning the bachelor's degree: lack of self-confidence and navigation of a complex academic system. Once these barriers have been dealt with, all that follows is easily manageable.

Financial aid is another important factor in student success. Prior to the implementation of the RN option, the schools of Education and Social Work had obtained a 30% tuition discount for professionals working full-time and attending classes part-time. A similar discount was negotiated for nursing students. In addition, many hospitals provided educational benefits that ranged from $1,000 per year to full payment of tuition and fees. The university and nursing financial aid advisers assisted those students who still had unmet financial need to obtain scholarships, service payback awards, and loans.

Between 1982 and 1987, a small amount of funding was received through the Special Needs Program of Title III of the Higher Education Act of 1965 for several projects, including the development of an evening and/or weekend program for the nurses. Weekend classes were not well attended by nurses, but the evening courses were a success. All required courses, liberal arts and nursing, except for three of the four sciences, were arranged to be offered in the late afternoon or evening.

The most important recruitment resources are the diploma and associate degree nursing programs in the immediate vicinity. Meetings of the advisers and administrators helped to coordinate the transition between the two levels. Course requirements, particularly in the sciences, have been strengthened and changed at one community college to facilitate transfer. A list of the Barry liberal arts and science requirements is in the advising computer at another community college. Yearly meetings of the Barry adviser with students in the diploma program have improved understanding and eased the transition between the two.

## FACULTY

The faculty members who teach the nurses are second in importance only to the RN adviser. The small number of students (9) at the beginning of the program did not require additional faculty. However, the need was great to meet the concerns of the faculty members who would be teaching the nurses. Faculty who would teach the nurses needed insight into and practice with the principles of adult education. Curricular questions had to be answered; admission, progression, and graduation requirements set; course sequencing determined; and roles clarified.

As the number of students increased and more faculty members were involved, some found more pleasure and success in teaching nurses than in teaching students in the basic option. New faculty who were hired for the RN option were expected to relate well with adults, have knowledge of adult education principles, be secure in their sense of self, and have solid clinical and educational expertise. In the end, however, faculty self-selected with more accuracy than was achieved by the best search committee.

## RECRUITMENT EFFORTS

Initially, there was no need for student recruitment because of the pool of displaced RN students. New students came to the program by word of mouth for several years. Active recruitment began in 1983 with a new program adviser. She used regularly scheduled recruitment and advisement sessions at about six major institutions in the area to identify and assist new students. Enrollment increased immediately from 30 to 42 and then to about 50, where it remained for several years. In 1985, the School of Nursing employed a former faculty member as director of enrollment management for all three undergraduate options. RN recruitment became more formalized and intense, with about 10 hospital visits per month. As a direct result of these activities, RN enrollment nearly tripled from 49 in fall 1985 to 138 in spring 1989.

## ADMISSIONS POLICIES

Admission requirements for the first RNs included Florida licensure, a 2.50 cumulative average, science courses taken no more than 10 years previously, three letters of recommendation, 2 years of full-time experience, scores from the licensure examination, and an interview with the dean at which time an essay would be written. In reality, only licensure and the 2.50 cumulative average were seriously considered in the admissions procedure. The essay and the experience requirements were removed after 4 years. From that time on, the interview served to impart information rather than being used for admission screening. In 1986, the science recency requirement was removed because of our understanding that practicing nurses were continually updating their science knowledge base. The following year, the requirement to present licensure examination scores was discontinued because the scores had never been considered seriously for admission.

Barry has rolling admissions: an admissions decision is made within 7 to 10 days after the application and required materials are received. Although originally there was an enrollment cap of 30 students, currently all qualified applicants are accepted. Students are admitted directly to the School of Nursing, and advising begins immediately. Because the majority of new students have prerequisites, liberal arts, and proficiency tests to complete, faculty have a two- to three-semester lead time for planning for nursing course enrollment.

## STUDENTS

The original enrollment of about 30 was arbitrarily chosen by faculty; it appeared to be satisfactory and was maintained for 6 years, from 1978 to 1984. Although 15 to 20 students were put on a waiting list, the faculty maintained enrollment at 30 until they had more experience with this new type of learner. In 1985 the number of RN students began to increase, and in 1986 a new goal of 50 RNs was set by the dean.

Originally enrolled students had diverse educational backgrounds and thus were placed at varying levels in the curriculum. Some were taking liberal arts, some taking proficiency and CLEP tests, and by 1979 the first five were taking nursing courses. In the group of 30 original RN students, the average age was 28.9 years; all except one were female; 22 were white non-Hispanic; and 4 were Hispanic. Records do not reveal the ethnic or racial heritage of the remaining four students. Nineteen had earned the associate degree in nursing; nine had earned a diploma; and two had both. Nineteen of the original 30 eventually graduated, taking from 1½ to 6½ years to complete their baccalaureate education. The average completion time for these students was 3 years. Of the 11 students who withdrew, about half (6) did so after the first year. The others withdrew in the second (4) or third years (1). Of the seven students whose reasons for withdrawing were known, two left for financial reasons, one changed to pre-med, two left for personal reasons, one was dissatisfied with the nursing program, and one left after being placed on academic probation.

The composition of the RN student body in fall 1988 was different in several ways from that of the original class of 1978. Although the ethnic ratios of the two groups remain about the same, the average age has increased from 29 to 36 years. The percentage of men has increased from 3 to 7, and the percentage of RNs with diplomas has increased from 30 to 45. Table 10.1 shows the comparison between the original and the most recent RN student bodies.

The first five students graduated in May 1980. The School of Nursing's annual report for that year reveals the following:

> The overall impression of this first group of five is that the BSN is a means to improve their employment status. Three of this group have immediate plans for graduate school and the other two will return to school after they have recouped their financial losses due to this educational sojourn (p. 2).

**TABLE 10.1. Comparison of Original and Current RN Classes of 1988**

| | 1978 n = 30 | | 1988 n = 123 | |
|---|---|---|---|---|
| | Number | Percent | Number | Percent |
| ETHNIC HERITAGE | | | | |
| White Non-Hispanic | 22 | 73 | 87 | 71 |
| Black | NA | | 21 | 17 |
| Hispanic | 4 | 13 | 13 | 11 |
| Asian | NA | | 2 | 2 |
| Unknown | 4 | 13 | 0 | 0 |
| SEX | | | | |
| Male | 1 | 3 | 8 | 7 |
| Female | 29 | 97 | 115 | 93 |
| ORIGINAL RN EDUCATION | | | | |
| Diploma | 9 | 30 | 55 | 45 |
| Associate Degree | 19 | 63 | 68 | 55 |
| Both | 2 | 7 | | |
| AGE | 28.9 years | | 36 years | |

In May 1983, a comprehensive follow-up survey was distributed to the 24 RNs who had completed the RN option during the first 4 years of the program. Participants were asked to evaluate both format and content of the option, as well as to provide biographical and descriptive information. The response rate was 70%.

Students ranged from 23 to 46 years of age on entering the program, with an average age of 30. They were predominantly female (96%), married or divorced (63%), white (96%), and graduates of an associate degree program in nursing (56%). "Professional development" was the reason cited most frequently for returning to school. Respondents were enrolled from 16 to 48 months, with an average length of 28 months to complete the program. Nurses spent an average of 3½ semesters as part-time students and 2½ as full-time students. Slightly more than half of the respondents (56%) lived in Broward, the county north of Miami, and commuted an average of 21 miles one way to attend Barry University.

Overall, RNs evaluated the RN option favorably but offered constructive suggestions. Nursing courses were predominantly rated as above average or superior. Respondents rated the program overall as above average (50%) or superior (31%). Ninety-four percent of the respondents indicated that they were encouraging other nurses to return to school and were recommending Barry University. Suggestions made by nurses included urging faculty to reconsider their teaching strategies and the selection of clinical experiences for students in this option.

## CURRICULUM

In 1978, the basic option (for generic students) contained 120 total credits, including natural sciences (24), composition and speech (9), philosophy and religion (9), behavioral and social sciences (12), nutrition (3), nursing (56), and electives (7). The nursing courses of 7 or 8 credits included the following: Nursing Process, Nursing Care of Mothers and Newborns, Nursing Care of Children, Nursing Care of Adults, Psychiatric Nursing, Community Health Nursing, and Nursing Leadership. Nursing courses of 1 or 2 credits included Trends and Issues, Nursing Research, and Health Assessment.

Four years after the initiation of the RN option, Barry revisited the liberal arts component of all curricula and revised the distribution requirements to be met by all who graduated from the university. For nursing, this change resulted in the reduction of credits in the natural sciences from 24 to 17 to accommodate the addition of 3 credits in statistics, 3 credits in computers, and 9 credits in the arts and humanities (in addition to the 9 in philosophy and religion). The 7 free elective credits were eliminated in order to maintain a total of 121 credits. At about the same time, the faculty made some minor changes in the nursing curriculum.

Initially, the basic option served as the model for the RN option. Nurses were required to obtain the same number and distribution of both nursing and liberal arts courses to earn the bachelor's degree as were students in the basic option. However, it was felt important to meet the needs of the nurse for different course times, a greater diversity of course locations, processes to validate previously learned content, and more independent learning methods to complete requirements. The decisions and accomplishments of the faculty to meet these needs are some of the major strengths of this option.

## LIBERAL ARTS AND PREREQUISITES

Of course, students could take all of the prerequisite, liberal arts and nursing courses at Barry to earn the degree, and a few chose to do this, particularly in the earlier years. However, most nurses took the liberal arts and prerequisite courses at a local community college or state university because of the lower costs and accessibility. To assist nurses who were interested in completing their degree at Barry to make the correct choices of courses at another institution, a course equivalent chart was developed. This sheet listed the Barry courses along the left margin and the course equivalents at three local community colleges and three nearby universities in the next six columns. Students could be confident that if they took a course on this list it would be accepted in transfer. However, there was one problem in our otherwise satisfying procedure.

University policy allowed the transfer of only 6 credits after an individual was admitted to Barry as a degree-seeking student. Thus, to give nurses the benefit of appropriate and accurate advising while they were taking additional courses elsewhere, we were admitting most nurses (if they were taking one or two Barry courses) as non-degree-seeking students. This resulted in a greatly diminished head count of students in the RN option because at that time non-degree-seeking students were listed as enrolled in the School of Arts and Sciences. The ability of the dean to justify the workload of the director was proportionately diminished.

The problem of head count was subsequently corrected, following meetings with the appropriate administrators, to reflect that nursing was the school of enrollment of the non-degree-seeking RN option students. Later the university allowed the School of Nursing to admit these students as degree-seeking, which in fact they were, and the 6-credit transferable limit was lifted. Although the classification of these students still provides us with occasional treasure hunts, by and large the numbers better reflect our actual head count.

Many of our RN students did not have transferable credit because they had attended a diploma program. These students were encouraged to earn credit by validating their learning in a variety of ways. Students were encouraged to take CLEP or proficiency tests. The university maintains an equivalency list for CLEP, which we distributed freely to nurses. We also advised them of the location and phone number of the nearest testing center.

The use of CLEP presented a problem that has since been solved. The university required that students present CLEP scores prior to the completion of 60 credits. Most nurses were being accepted with that many credits or more from their previous degree. Although the number of students who sought CLEP credit was small, the 60-credit rule was waived. However, students are encouraged to earn CLEP credit within the first semester of enrollment.

Barry has long had a policy of allowing students to earn credit for courses by taking a proficiency or teacher-made cumulative test, usually the final. These tests were available for courses for which there was no CLEP test: they were taken for credit/no credit only, and could not be repeated. The RN option adviser made contact with the appropriate faculty members, who prepared study guides or augmented syllabi from which students could prepare. Proficiency tests and the preparation materials were formally evaluated by each student who used them, and the evaluation was shared with the course faculty member. Thus, students were able to earn credit for all science, liberal arts, and prerequisite courses through the use of transfer, CLEP, or proficiency tests.

One additional method to earn credit for liberal arts courses taken in diploma programs was recently accepted. Through conversations with students it became apparent that although some courses had been taken in a diploma program, they had been taught by a faculty member who presented the same course while teaching full-time at the local community college. It appeared that the diploma school course was essentially the same as that for which credit was earned by associate degree students. Thus, if the nurse could obtain a letter indicating that the faculty member had taught the same course at the community college, the course was accepted for credit without the necessity of validation by test.

For nurses earning the BSN, the Barry Division of Adult and Continuing Education (ACE) is an important source for the liberal arts requirements. Courses are taught once a week in 4-hour blocks during 10-week sessions continuing throughout the year. They are offered every weekday evening, including Fridays, during the day, and on Saturday mornings. Sites for classes—police stations, hospitals, community colleges, office buildings, naval bases, and various other locations—are located in many counties in South Florida. Some courses are audiotaped, and students can complete course requirements by using the tapes at home. Tuition for ACE courses is about one half of that on the main campus. Coordination between the RN option adviser and the staff at ACE often led to initiating courses at a time and place attractive to nurses earning the BSN.

Another method to earn credit that meets the needs of the adult learner is to take courses by correspondence. The Florida state university system provides for enrollment in numerous correspondence courses, which allows students to complete the learning and validation of that learning in an independent mode. Students are enrolled with the signature of their adviser at Barry and receive the guidebook for the course. They may be required to complete 10 to 20 written lessons, one or several papers, or one or several tests (proctored at Barry). The student has full control of the time and place of learning. The course is fully acceptable in transfer, as is any other course taken in one of the state universities.

## NURSING

As with the liberal arts, nurses were originally required to demonstrate proficiency by test or to take the same nursing courses as students in the basic option. Nurses were invited to demonstrate proficiency in five lower-level nursing courses through teacher-made written and clinical examinations, earning 30 credits. Prior to beginning the first examination, students were required to have completed 7 credits at Barry (reduced to 6 credits in 1982), 4 of which must have been in physiology (advanced normal). In the first year, 195 nursing credit hours were generated through proficiency examinations. Of the 30 examinations administered, students successfully passed 25. Initially, the sequence of proficiency tests and courses was less prescribed. Progression later became more orderly, and enrollment in the required nursing courses was preceded by successful completion of all theoretical and clinical proficiency testing for the lower-level nursing courses.

In 1984, the NLN Mobility Profile II was carefully examined at Barry and chosen to replace teacher-made proficiencies. Shortly thereafter, the NLN achievement test, Nursing Care of Adults in Special Care Units, was added to the Mobility Profile. In 1985, 109 nurses took one or more of these tests, with a few failures in Care of the Client During Childbearing, Care of the Child, and Care of the Client with a Mental Disorder. Most or all passed Care of the Adult Client and Nursing Care of Adults in Special Care Units. In 1985, the overall passing rate on the NLN Mobility Profile was 72% (on the first sitting). Students were allowed to repeat the test once.

Also at about this time, clinical testing for nurses was discontinued as a routine for students in the RN option. Only rarely did a nurse fail these examinations, which were extremely time-consuming for faculty members. However, clinical testing could be required for students who had not actively practiced clinical nursing in 3 years or those who demonstrated low scores on the NLN Mobility Profile or achievement tests.

RN option students were required to enroll in Health Assessment, Trends and Issues in Nursing, Nursing Research, Community Health Nursing, Nursing Management, and one other clinical course of their choice, usually the course in which they were least able to demonstrate proficiency. All of these courses were taken with students in the basic option. The nurses were viewed positively by both faculty and basic-option students, and their contributions in courses as well as individually were valued. As they moved into the required nursing clinical courses, nurses began to experience a sense of belonging to the Barry University School of Nursing. For example, in 1981, nine nurses participated in pinning and two more attended as audience.

During the curriculum revision of 1983, content in the trends and assessment courses was integrated, and therefore these courses no longer existed as separate entities. In response to the necessity of making this content available to the RN option student, a "bridge" course, Processes in Nursing, was designed and offered for the first time, replacing the previously required clinical nursing course elective. Processes in Nursing (7 credits) addressed the adult learning needs of this group and the process threads unique to the Barry curriculum. The course description stated: "Introduction and overview of the philosophy, concepts, and theories which form the conceptual framework. Concepts of nursing process, communication, change, teaching-learning, research, and professionalism. Skills in health assessment presented and practiced." It was team-taught, and the evaluations were overwhelmingly positive, perhaps partly because this course established students as a class of bonded individuals. Sixteen nurses took the course in both the first and second years. The prerequisite for enrollment in the bridge course was completion of all four sciences, 60 credits of coursework, and the NLN Mobility Profile II and NLN achievement tests.

Three years later, it became evident that the diversity and amount of content in Processes of Nursing had become overwhelming to nurses and the faculty team. In addition, students appeared to need more content in role theory, interpersonal relations, and group processes than they were receiving. Therefore, the course was divided into Professional Processes (4 credits), Processes of Interpersonal Communication (2 credits), Group and Organizational Dynamics (2 credits), Professional Role Seminar (2 credits), and Health Assessment (3 credits). Each course is taught by an individual faculty member under the guidance of the RN option director.

Although 30 nurses were enrolled during the first year at various stages of the program, only 4 or 5 RN students were taking clinical courses at any one time. Thus, there were not enough nurses for a separate section of these courses. Although there appeared to be mutual benefit to all students in putting RNs together with the basic-option students, in fact the benefit was more in favor of the generic students than of the nurses. RN students had nursing experience from which to contribute to class discussions and were more willing to participate in seminar activities than generic students were. Generic students frequently depended on RN students rather than faculty for help in the clinical area, sometimes impeding RN students' learning.

Finally, by 1985, all-RN sections of community health and nursing management were offered for the first time. This change was a result of evaluating the different supervision needs of nurses, the necessity to use different learning exercises and clinical assignments to attain the objectives for both types of students, and a sufficient increase in the number of nurses to support a separate section. Continuing evaluation by faculty and RN option students supports placing nurses in a separate track from students in the basic option.

During the past 10 years, nurses have requested that faculty evaluate various other tests and methods to validate previous learning without repeating tested content. Nurses in critical care and other specialties suggested that the test to earn certification be accepted in lieu of the NLN Mobility Profile or achievement tests. From time to time, specific courses taught at community colleges, such as critical care and community health, have been evaluated for transferability in place of required courses. Faculty members are examining the possibility of allowing RN students to develop a portfolio to demonstrate learning attained through experience in community health nursing and/or nursing management. All possibilities are open to evaluation in an effort to reduce the replication of learning.

Additional adjustments have been made in the RN option for unique groups of students. For example, nurses who had previously earned a non-nursing bachelor's degree, including the bachelor of professional studies from Barry's ACE Division, were not required to match, course for course, the university distribution requirements. With the exception of the sciences, statistics, philosophy or religion, and biomedical ethics, the faculty believed that these students had already achieved a liberal education. They needed only to complete the above courses and nursing.

Another unique group included nurses whose immediate goal was the master's degree in nursing. These students were carefully evaluated for admission to the RN-to-MSN option, allowing them to earn 12 graduate credits in place of similar undergraduate courses, thus preventing unnecessary duplication of content. These students are awarded the bachelor's degree in nursing, but they are required to earn only 33 more credits (instead of the usual 45) to complete the master's degree.

## OUTREACH

In implementing an RN option, the question of outreach must be considered. Two years ago, off-campus sites for the RN option at Barry were first explored. A preliminary needs study was initiated in the Indian River/Ft. Pierce area, 100 miles north of Miami. Need and interest appeared to exist. Visits to Naples/Ft. Meyers, 100 miles west of Miami, were also conducted. However, the first off-campus site was in Palm Beach, 60 miles north of Miami, where yet another university program for nurses had closed and Barry had again been invited to assist the stranded students to complete their degree work. About 30 students are currently enrolled at ACE and nursing courses in this area, and because there is a great amount of interest, new nursing course sequences will begin about every other semester at this site.

The initiation of outreach programs is being carefully evaluated and planned. Regional, state, and professional accrediting bodies provide specific guidance for these sites. There appear to be sufficient students for the program in Palm Beach. Resources, particularly faculty, library, and clinical, are being measured very carefully. Support from the nursing community at the outreach site must be deep. A decision must include thoughtful choice of the model of outreach, whether a continuing program or a one-time program.

## SUMMARY

Our experience at Barry of participating in the continuing educational development of nurses in Dade, Broward, and Palm Beach counties has been a strongly positive one. We began quickly and conservatively but have moved steadily toward a liberal, although controlled, RN option. The greatest strength of the option has been and continues to be the advisers and faculty members who enjoy working with adults. The ability of the faculty to be open to challenge, to hear requests for change, to evaluate change in the light of balancing individual student concerns with institutional and program integrity, and to rapidly implement decisions for change has made our RN option a positive experience for nurses.

So Barry continues the process of developing and expanding the RN option as we begin our second decade of serving these unique students. Aggressive recruitment is no longer necessary: our graduates have become our best recruiters.

# Appendix A:
## Essentials of College and University Education for Professional Nursing: Final Report

**TABLE OF CONTENTS**

# NATIONAL PANEL FOR ESSENTIALS OF COLLEGE AND UNIVERSITY EDUCATION FOR PROFESSIONAL NURSING

*CHAIR*     Edward H. Jennings, PhD
President
The Ohio State University

*MEMBERS*   Patricia Benner, PhD, RN
Associate Professor of Nursing
University of California-San Francisco

Mary Champagne, PhD, RN
Assistant Professor of Nursing
University of North Carolina at Chapel Hill

Joyce C. Clifford, MSN, RN
Vice President of Nursing
Beth Israel Hospital, Boston

Sheldon S. King
Executive Vice President and Director*
Stanford University Medical Center

Julia A. Lane, PhD, RN
Dean and Professor of Nursing
Loyola University of Chicago

Jo McNeil, MN, RN
Director of Nursing Research*
Seattle-King County Department of Public Health

L. Jackson Newell, PhD
Dean of Liberal Education
University of Utah

Dorothy L. Powell, EdD, RN
Chairperson and Associate Professor of Nursing
Norfolk State University

Neal A. Vanselow, MD
Vice President for Health Sciences
University of Minnesota

*Project Staff*  Betty M. Johnson, PhD, RN
Project Director

Barbara K. Redman, PhD, RN
Executive Director

Karla J. Cowell, MA
Staff Associate

*Position when selected for the Panel.

# ESSENTIALS OF COLLEGE AND UNIVERSITY EDUCATION FOR PROFESSIONAL NURSING
### Report to the Membership of AACN
### October 1986

In 1984, the American Association of Colleges of Nursing received a grant from the Pew Memorial Trust to define education for professional nursing. The proposal was based on recommendations in the Institute of Medicine Study on Nursing and Nursing Education (1983) and the Report of the National Commission on Nursing (1983). The project, entitled "Essentials of College and University Education for Professional Nursing," was directed by a national panel of representatives from the nursing, health care, and higher education communities. Three work groups assisted with the project. Although there have been previous attempts at the national level to deal with specific issues related to nursing education, the current project represents the first comprehensive national effort to define the essential knowledge, practice, and values that the baccalaureate nurse should possess.

**The panel recommends that every program preparing nurses for the first professional degree include educational experiences for each of the essentials.** The depth of exposure and the method of providing the education for the essentials will vary from program to program. In addition, most programs will include education beyond the essentials based on characteristics of the university or college in which the program is located, the student body, the community, and health care institutions and agencies where students learn clinical judgment and practice skills. Although the essential knowledge, practice, and values are presented in separate sections of the report, the panel recognizes that the essentials are interrelated parts of the entire educational process.

The task of the panel and work groups was to define the essential components rather than the total education of the professional nurse. Education prior to college or university, for example, is not included. **The panel recommends that each program establish requirements for admission including those related to general education.**

Before presenting the essentials, the context of nursing and its effect on education and the socialization of the student into nursing are discussed.

## The Context of Nursing and Its Effect on Education

The role of the nurse has expanded considerably in the past 20 years matching the pace of change in the health care system. Rapid changes in health care, especially those related to age groups, care settings, and technology, require that the professional nurse has an up-to-date knowledge and practice base, the motivation and skills for life-long learning, and the ability to translate new knowledge and skills into health care for individuals, families, groups and communities. These changes have implications for curricular content, clinical learning sites, new areas of specialized knowledge, and changed responsibilities. The following illustrate the effects that some changes have had on the context of nursing.

A shift from retrospective reimbursement to prospective payment in health care has led to early discharge and the need for nurses to administer complex care in homes and alternative health settings. Home care of the acutely and chronically ill and the establishment of hospices have increased the need for the delivery of nursing care in community settings. A redistribution of power has modified the roles of nurses and physicians and the missions of health care agencies. In addition, consumers are assuming more decision-making responsibility for their health. Technological advances present ethical dilemmas such as the right to die, allocation of donor organs, and the balance between high technology and high touch. The cultural diversity of consumers and the variability in their knowledge of health care are factors that have increased the need for health care advocacy.

Professional nurses, who are primary health providers, engage in a broad range of health promotion and teaching activities and coordinate care in every sector of the health care system. Nurses have major roles in wellness and health promotion, in acute care, and in long-term care for chronic illness. Each of these areas is discussed briefly.

*Wellness and Health Promotion*  The nurse, who has direct contact with people at all levels of health and in diverse settings, has a key role in health teaching and health promotion. These two functions are likely to expand in scope and significance as life style and stress are implicated in the development of diseases such as stroke, heart disease, and cancer. Nurses are becoming increasingly involved in community wellness efforts focused on health education, life style change, early childhood health, and stress-management. Nurses assist people by helping them learn to deal with daily health problems. In addition, many nursing interventions focus on identifying and decreasing health risks.

*Acute Care*  The complexity and intrusiveness of highly technical health care has increased the acuity levels of hospitalized patients/clients* and expanded the diagnostic-monitoring activities of the nurse. The nurse is faced with the need for immediate responses to unstable conditions and greater participation in decisions about life and death. The intensity of

---

*Throughout the document, patient/client refers to individuals, families, groups, and communities.

disease conditions along with abbreviated hospitalizations requires the nurse to provide extensive support and education.

*Long-Term Care for Chronic Illness*  The number of chronically ill and injured individuals has increased the need for rehabilitation and follow-up care. Increases in stress-related chronic illness, survival rates of people with major injuries, and an aging population require efforts to support and teach self-care to individuals and families in order to achieve maximum functioning. Meeting these health care needs falls primarily in nursing's domain.

The diversity and complexity of nursing practice in today's health care field makes it necessary to prepare nurses who can think critically and creatively and who have a sound education in nursing science, related sciences, and the humanities.

**The panel recommends that the essential knowledge, practice, and values presented in this document be interpreted in light of the roles and responsibilities discussed above.**

## Socialization

Socialization is a largely subconscious process by which an individual acquires the attributes associated with a profession. Through the socialization process, the student develops a sense of identity and commitment to the profession by internalizing the norms, values, knowledge, skills, and behaviors shared by members of that profession.

The socialization process results in the following outcomes:

1. A linkage between the individual's motivation for entering nursing and the development of professional behavior.
2. A nursing perspective and related critical-thinking and problem-solving skills.
3. Mastery of the knowledge and skills of the profession.
4. Internalization of the values, traditions, and obligations of the professional.
5. Identification with and commitment to the profession.

The student enters the college or university with knowledge, skills, and values that are expanded and modified through the educational process. Faculty serve as socializing agents through modeling and teaching the professional role; demonstrating mastery of nursing knowledge, skills, and behaviors; and exhibiting commitment to values, traditions, obligations, and concerns of the profession. These socialization strategies are a planned part of the educational process.

Being successful in the nursing role and adopting attributes of the profession help the student identify with and gain commitment to the profession. As a sense of personal worth develops, the student moves from mere enactment of the role to becoming a professional nurse.

# LIBERAL EDUCATION

In 1984 and 1985, three national panels recommended improvements for the undergraduate curriculum, especially in liberal education (Association of American Colleges, 1985; National Institute of Education, 1984; and National Endowment for the Humanities, 1984). **We recommend that the education of the professional nurse reflect the spirit of these reports so that the graduate will exhibit qualities of mind and character that are necessary to live a free and fulfilling life, act in the public interest locally and globally, and contribute to health care improvements and the nursing profession.** The aim of education is to prepare a fully-functioning human being. A major nursing function is to enhance the well-being of others, therefore, the nurse must have the educational foundation to foster personal well-being and continuing growth.

Knowledge is neither the exclusive province of the experts in an academic discipline nor limited to a specific set of courses. The whole academic community shares responsibility for the education of the student. Knowledge acquired at the college or university level builds on previous experience and learning and is enhanced by collaboration among faculty from many disciplines. The liberally educated person who is prepared in this manner can responsibly challenge the status quo and anticipate and adapt to change.

**We recommend that the education of the professional nurse ensure the ability to:**

1. Write, read, and speak English clearly and effectively in order to acquire knowledge, convey and discuss ideas, evaluate information, and think critically.
2. Think analytically and reason logically using verifiable information and past experience in order to select or create solutions to problems.
3. Understand a second language, at least at an elementary level, in order to widen access to the diversity of world cultures.
4. Understand other cultural traditions in order to gain a perspective on personal values and the similarities and differences among individuals and groups.
5. Use mathematical concepts, interpret quantitative data, and use computers and other information technology in order to analyze problems and develop positions that depend on numbers and statistics.
6. Use concepts from the behavioral and biological sciences in order to understand oneself and one's relationships with other people and to comprehend the nature and function of communities.
7. Understand the physical world and its interrelationship with human activity in order to make decisions that are based on

scientific evidence and responsive to the values and interests of the individual and society.

8. Comprehend life and time from historical and contemporary perspectives and draw from past experiences to influence the present and future.

9. Gain a perspective on social, political, and economic issues for resolving societal and professional problems.

10. Comprehend the meaning of human spirituality in order to recognize the relationship of beliefs to culture, behavior, health, and healing.

11. Appreciate the role of the fine and performing arts in stimulating individual creativity, expressing personal feelings and emotions, and building a sense of the commonality of human experience.

12. Understand the nature of human values and develop a personal philosophy in order to make ethical judgments in both personal and professional life.

Professors of nursing, like all faculty, must help shape and actively support the liberal education requirements of their colleges and universities. Nursing faculty are responsible for integrating knowledge from the liberal arts and sciences into professional nursing education and practice. Liberally educated nurses make informed and responsible ethical choices and help shape the future of society as well as the nursing profession.

## VALUES AND PROFESSIONAL BEHAVIORS

College and university education for professional nursing includes processes that foster the development of values, attitudes, personal qualities, and professional behaviors. Values are defined as beliefs or ideals to which an individual is committed and which guide behavior. Values are reflected in attitudes, personal qualities, and consistent patterns of behavior. Attitudes are inclinations or dispositions to respond positively or negatively to a person, object, or situation, while personal qualities are innate or learned attributes of an individual. Professional behaviors reflect the individual's commitment to specific values.

Nursing has been described as a cultural paradox. The professional nurse must adopt contemporary characteristics such as independence, assertiveness, self-esteem, and confidence as well as those of a more traditional nature such as compassion, acceptance, consideration, and kindness. Adoption of the essential values leads the nurse to a sense of commitment and social responsibility, a sensitivity and responsiveness to the needs of others, and a responsibility for oneself and one's actions.

**We recommend that the following seven values are essential for the**

**professional nurse.** Examples of attitudes, personal qualities, and professional behaviors are included that reflect a commitment to one or more of these values.

| ESSENTIAL VALUES* | EXAMPLES OF ATTITUDES AND PERSONAL QUALITIES | EXAMPLES OF PROFESSIONAL BEHAVIORS |
|---|---|---|
| **1. ALTRUISM** Concern for the welfare of others. | Caring Commitment Compassion Generosity Perseverance | Gives full attention to the patient/client when giving care. Assists other personnel in providing care when they are unable to do so. Expresses concern about social trends and issues that have implications for health care. |
| **2. EQUALITY** Having the same rights, privileges, or status. | Acceptance Assertiveness Fairness Self-esteem Tolerance | Provides nursing care based on the individual's needs irrespective of personal characteristics.** Interacts with other providers in a non-discriminatory manner. Expresses ideas about the improvement of access to nursing and health care. |
| **3. ESTHETICS** Qualities of objects, events, and persons that provide satisfaction. | Appreciation Creativity Imagination Sensitivity | Adapts the environment so it is pleasing to the patient/client. Creates a pleasant work environment for self and others. Presents self in a manner that promotes a positive image of nursing. |
| **4. FREEDOM** Capacity to exercise choice. | Confidence Hope Independence Openness Self-direction Self-discipline | Honors individuals's right to refuse treatment. Supports the rights of other providers to suggest alternatives to the plan of care. Encourages open discussion of controversial issues in the profession. |

---

* The values are listed in alphabetic rather than priority order.

**From CODE FOR NURSES, American Nurses' Association, 1976.

| 5. HUMAN DIGNITY Inherent worth and uniqueness of an individual. | Consideration Empathy Humaneness Kindness Respectfulness Trust | Safeguards the individual's right to privacy. Addresses individuals as they prefer to be addressed. Maintains confidentiality of patients/clients and staff. Treats others with respect regardless of background. |
| --- | --- | --- |
| 6. JUSTICE Upholding moral and legal principles. | Courage Integrity Morality Objectivity | Acts as a health care advocate. Allocates resources fairly. Reports incompetent, unethical, and illegal practice objectively and factually.* |
| 7. TRUTH Faithfulness to fact or reality. | Accountability Authenticity Honesty Inquisitiveness Rationality Reflectiveness | Documents nursing care accurately and honestly. Obtains sufficient data to make sound judgments before reporting infractions of organizational policies. Participates in professional efforts to protect the public from misinformation about nursing. |

The professional nurse assigns priorities to these values within specific decision-making contexts in the application of essential knowledge and practice. The nurse, guided by these values, attitudes, and personal qualities, demonstrates ethical professional behavior with patients/ clients, colleagues, and others in providing safe, humanistic care focused on health and quality of life. Values, attitudes, personal qualities, and consistent patterns of behavior begin to develop early in life, but also are fostered and facilitated by selected educational strategies and the process of socialization to the profession.

## KNOWLEDGE AND PROFESSIONAL NURSING PRACTICE

Professional nursing practice is based on liberal and professional knowledge, clinical and cognitive skills, and the value system of the individual. Professional nursing encompasses the care of individuals, families, groups, and communities as well as health teaching and health promotion.

Nursing practice is a type of knowledge, an application of knowledge,

---

*From CODE FOR NURSES, American Nurses' Association, 1976.

and a way of knowing. The application of clinical knowledge requires judgment and innovation. Clinical knowledge may be formalized into theory as a result of systematically studying nursing practice.

Nursing students must develop the knowledge and skill essential for clinical judgment in diverse contexts of nursing practice. Therefore, it is important that students learn strategies for systematic data collection, assessment, implementation, and evaluation of nursing care. Clinical judgments are made and nursing interventions are selected and administered based on data collection and assessment.

Clinical judgment is the process of translating knowledge and observation into a plan of nursing action and the implementation of that plan for the benefit of the patient/client. The clinical judgment of the professional nurse focuses on the outcomes of nursing and health care. These outcomes include staying healthy, avoiding illness, increasing well-being, decreasing symptoms of illness and discomfort, getting well, and coping with irreversible changes and death. Astute clinical judgment is essential for the diagnostic and monitoring functions of professional practice and is verified by successful health care outcomes.

The nurse functions in a variety of settings and confronts various human responses and a wide range of ages, cultures, health beliefs, and individual expectations in the practice of professional nursing. Clinical judgments permeate this entire practice. The nature and scope of clinical judgments distinguish the practice of the professional nurse from others who may participate in nursing activities or carry out certain nursing procedures. Clinical judgment in unstructured settings and in situations with unpredictable outcomes are specific responsibilities of the professional nurse and, therefore, are emphasized in college and university education for nursing.

Nursing intervention includes cognitive, psychosocial, and psychomotor skills based on the nursing plan of care or the plans of other health care professionals. Intervention provides additional opportunities for data collection. Examples of nursing interventions and clinical skills with minimal levels of achievement essential for the new graduate of a professional nursing program are presented in the appendix of this report.

**We recommend that programs preparing nurses for the first professional degree include educational experiences for each of the following essentials. We further recommend that graduates of professional nursing programs possess the nursing interventions and clinical skills necessary to make clinical judgments** (See examples in Appendix A).

This section of the document is organized according to three major roles of the nurse: provider of care, coordinator of care, and member of a profession. The provider of care section is further organized according to the nursing process.

## PROVIDER OF CARE

The professional nurse provides nursing care to individuals, families, groups, and communities along a continuum of health, illness, and disability in multiple settings. The nurse is concerned with assessing health, illness, and the response to disease as well as the relationships among these three. Nursing requires skills for collecting clinical data about health, illness, symptoms, expected and preferred modes of treatment, recovery, and the patient's/client's interpretation of these states. Systematic assessment, which includes communication and planning skills, helps ensure that nursing care goals are congruent with the patient's/client's needs and preferences.

Nursing interventions are delivered in a variety of settings, cover a broad range of intents, and require a commitment to caring. These interventions require clinical judgment skills; diagnostic and monitoring skills; and helping, coaching, teaching, counseling, and communication skills. Nursing interventions focus on preventing illness; promoting health; and maximizing physical, functional, and psychosocial status. In addition to direct intervention, nursing is concerned with marshalling appropriate family, community, and professional resources to augment self-care and nursing care, as well as collaborating with and assisting other health care providers in the delivery of care.

The primary intents of evaluation are to ensure the adequacy of the care plan in meeting goals, improve the process of intervention, and develop nursing knowledge. Evaluative clinical judgments are built on nursing assessment skills and related knowledge; planning skills enable the nurse to modify the plan of care and the process of care delivery.

1.  **KNOWLEDGE NEEDED TO DETERMINE HEALTH STATUS AND HEALTH NEEDS BASED ON THE INTERPRETATION OF HEALTH-RELATED DATA.**
    a.  Theories and models that guide nursing practice.
    b.  Nursing process.
    c.  System of classification for nursing diagnosis.
    d.  Data collection tools and techniques of assessment for individuals, families, groups, and communities.
    e.  Characteristics, concepts, and processes related to individuals including anatomy and physiology; physical and psychosocial growth and development; pathophysiology and psychopathology; and cultural and spiritual beliefs and practices related to health, illness, birth, and death and dying.
    f.  Characteristics, concepts, and processes related to families and groups including family development, structure, and function; family communication patterns and decision-making structures; family and group dynamics and behavior; and family and group dysfunction.

g. Characteristics, concepts, and processes related to communities including epidemiology, risk factors and their implications for selected populations, resources and resource assessment techniques, environmental factors, and social organization.
h. Distinctions and relationships between health status, health-seeking behaviors, illness experiences, and disease processes.
i. Diagnoses, therapies, and treatments of patients/clients to whom care is being given.

**1.1 CLINICAL JUDGMENTS AND RELATED SKILLS** needed to select and obtain health data in collaboration with individuals, their families, and other health care professionals.
a. Take patient/client history to obtain physical, psychosocial, cultural, familial, occupational, and environmental information.
b. Perform basic examination to identify health status and monitor for change.

**1.2 CLINICAL JUDGMENTS AND RELATED SKILLS** needed to make nursing diagnoses based on health-related data.
a. Analyze health data of individuals and their families.
b. Interpret health-related data.
c. Document nursing diagnoses.

**2. KNOWLEDGE NEEDED TO FORMULATE GOALS AND A PLAN OF CARE IN COLLABORATION WITH PATIENTS/ CLIENTS AND OTHER HEALTH CARE PROFESSIONALS.**
a. The dynamics of the nurse-patient/nurse-client relationship.
b. Principles of prevention from health promotion to health restoration.
c. Interventions to promote and restore health, prevent illness, and provide rehabilitation.
d. Interventions to support the individual and family during life stages and experiences including death and dying.
e. Relationship between the nursing plan of care, the therapeutic regimen, and the plans of other health care professionals.
f. Criteria for setting priorities.
g. Strategies for coordinating care resources.
h. Strategies for discharge planning.

**2.1 CLINICAL JUDGMENTS AND RELATED SKILLS** needed to establish a plan of care based on the nursing diagnoses and patient/ client preferences in collaboration with the patient/client and other health care providers.
a. Identify goals and select interventions.
b. Coordinate care plan with patient/client goals.

c. Monitor consistency between the nursing plan of care and the plans and intents of other health care professionals.

d. Communicate plan to nurses and other health care providers.

3. **KNOWLEDGE NEEDED TO IMPLEMENT THE PLAN OF CARE.**

a. Health practices and behaviors related to cultures, belief systems, and the environment.

b. Patterns and modes of communication.

c. Rights and responsibilities of people related to health care.

d. Physical, emotional, and cultural responses to illness and disease, such as pain, dyspnea, anxiety, and loneliness.

e. Biological, psychosocial, and spiritual aspects of nursing interventions.

f. Principles and theories of factors that maintain or restore health such as nutrition, rest, and exercise.

g. Physiological and psychological aspects of the healing process.

h. Properties, effects, and principles underlying the use and administration of therapeutic agents including pharmaceuticals, blood products, and oxygen.

i. Principles of asepsis.

j. Theories and strategies of stress management and crisis intervention.

k. Framework for ethical decision making.

l. Legal parameters of nursing practice and health care.

m. Interdisciplinary resources and relationships.

**3.1 CLINICAL JUDGMENTS AND RELATED SKILLS** needed to assist the individual to meet basic physiological needs in any state of health or setting.

a. Promote a safe, comfortable environment conducive to the optimal health and dignity of the individual.

b. Assist individual to meet nutritional and fluid and electrolyte needs.

c. Assist individual to meet elimination needs.

d. Assist individual to meet oxygenation needs.

e. Assist individual to attain adequate activity, comfort, rest, and sleep.

f. Assist individual with activities of daily living.

g. Promote rehabilitation.

h. Provide initial intervention for selected emergencies.

**3.2 CLINICAL JUDGMENTS AND RELATED SKILLS** needed to assist the individual and family to address psycho-social and spiritual concerns related to health care needs, for example, death and dying, stress, body image, self-esteem, and sexuality.

a. Promote psychosocial well-being.
b. Promote the adequacy of sensory stimulation.
c. Foster individual and family growth during developmental transitions.
d. Promote individual and family integrity and autonomy.

**3.3 CLINICAL JUDGMENTS AND RELATED SKILLS** needed to assist other health care providers to carry out the health care plan.
a. Administer medications and treatments.
b. Assist nurse clinician, nurse practitioner, or physician with frequently performed procedures.
c. Monitor responses to treatments and communicate them to other health care professionals.

**3.4 CLINICAL JUDGMENTS AND RELATED SKILLS** needed to assist the individual and family to identify ethical and legal issues that affect health needs, such as right to die or refuse treatment, informed consent, and use of least restrictive restraints.
a. Interpret health rights to patients/clients.
b. Recognize ethical and legal concerns.
c. Use interdisciplinary resources to address ethical and legal concerns.

**3.5 CLINICAL JUDGMENTS AND RELATED SKILLS** needed to document patient/client information and communicate to other nurses and health care providers.
a. Use standard terminology and form.
b. Provide concise, pertinent, and complete data.

**4. KNOWLEDGE NEEDED TO DEFINE LEARNING NEEDS OF INDIVIDUALS AND GROUPS RELATED TO HEALTH.**
a. Developmental norms and situation variables affecting learning.
b. Principles of learning.
c. Principles, methods, strategies and outcomes related to health teaching.

**4.1 CLINICAL JUDGMENTS AND RELATED SKILLS** needed to educate individuals and small groups concerning the promotion, maintenance, and restoration of health.
a. Develop teaching plans for common situations incorporating short and long-range goals of individuals, families, and groups.
b. Implement the teaching plan using various teaching and learning strategies.
c. Evaluate learning outcomes.

5. **KNOWLEDGE NEEDED TO EVALUATE PATIENT/CLIENT RESPONSES TO THERAPEUTIC INTERVENTIONS.**
   a. Methods for measuring goal attainment.
   b. Methods for evaluating the quality of nursing practice.

5.1 **CLINICAL JUDGMENTS AND RELATED SKILLS** needed to evaluate the quality of care in terms of patient/client understanding and satisfaction, health and disease states, illness experiences, and cost effectiveness.
   a. Compare expected and achieved outcomes of care.
   b. Identify reasons for deviation from plan of care.
   c. Alter plan of care and/or expected outcomes.

6. **KNOWLEDGE NEEDED TO PROVIDE CARE FOR MULTIPLE\* PATIENTS/CLIENTS.**
   a. A model for the delivery of nursing care.
   b. Characteristics, trends, and issues of health care delivery.
   c. Basis for determining priorities in care situations including principles of triage.
   d. Decision-making processes within organizations.
   e. Principles of delegation, supervision, and collaboration.

6.1 **CLINICAL JUDGMENTS AND RELATED SKILLS** needed to provide direct care to multiple\* patients/clients in acute, long term, and community settings.
   a. Identify priorities and make judgments concerning the needs of a group of patients/clients.
   b. Implement multiple plans of care.

7. **KNOWLEDGE NEEDED TO USE AN ANALYTICAL APPROACH AS THE BASIS FOR DECISION MAKING IN PRACTICE.**
   a. Nursing process.
   b. The scientific method.
   c. A conceptual model of nursing practice as a means of planning care and solving clinical problems.
   d. Sources of information including clinical data and research findings.

7.1 **CLINICAL JUDGMENTS AND RELATED SKILLS** needed to use clinical data and research findings as a basis for practice.
   a. Analyze published and unpublished clinical studies.
   b. Identify areas or problems for study.
   c. Participate in evaluation of nursing practice activities.

---

\*Three or more

## COORDINATOR OF CARE

As the coordinator of health care, the nurse is involved in organizing and facilitating the delivery of comprehensive, efficient, and appropriate service to individuals, families, groups, and communities. The coordinator of care is aware of other providers' services, the complexity of human and material resources, and the importance of collaboration with patients/clients, their support systems, and a variety of providers. During the planning and coordinating of care, the nurse demonstrates the ability to conceptualize the total continuing health needs of the patient/client and the impact of critical issues including legal and ethical aspects of care. Planning and coordinating skills, though fundamental to nursing, require ongoing practice and experience.

8. **KNOWLEDGE NEEDED TO COORDINATE HUMAN AND MATERIAL RESOURCES FOR PROVISION OF CARE.**
   a. Theories of leadership, decision making, motivation, and management.
   b. Group process as a means for achieving mutual goals.
   c. Human and material resources for providing quality care.

8.1 **CLINICAL JUDGMENTS AND RELATED SKILLS** needed to promote positive work group relationships that facilitate identification and attainment of nursing care goals.
   a. Use leadership skills to meet goals and enhance quality of nursing care.
   b. Identify change strategies appropriate to goal attainment.

8.2 **CLINICAL JUDGMENTS AND RELATED SKILLS** needed to guide and supervise nursing care.
   a. Assist nursing personnel to implement nursing care plan.
   b. Supervise implementation of care plan.

8.3 **CLINICAL JUDGMENTS AND RELATED SKILLS** needed to participate in evaluation of group members according to established protocol and using predetermined criteria.
   a. Evaluate the care administered by other group members.
   b. Facilitate changes in group member's performance to improve care.

9. **KNOWLEDGE NEEDED TO COLLABORATE WITH PATIENTS/ CLIENTS, CO-WORKERS, AND OTHERS FOR PROVISION OF CARE.**
   a. Patterns and modes of effective communication and collaboration.
   b. Strategies for initiating change in behavior patterns.

c. Effects of system organization on social interaction within the system.

d. Structure and function of the health care delivery system and relationships between the system and other social systems.

**9.1 CLINICAL JUDGMENTS AND RELATED SKILLS** needed to collaborate with patients/clients, co-workers, and others to improve health care for individuals, families, and groups.

a. Seek opportunities to work with patients/clients and other health care providers to improve health care.

b. Promote and participate in interdisciplinary health planning within and among health care systems.

**10. KNOWLEDGE NEEDED TO REFER INDIVIDUALS AND THEIR FAMILIES TO APPROPRIATE SOURCES OF ASSISTANCE.**

a. Referral process.

b. Community services, institutional resources, and the roles of other health care providers.

b. Interdependence of the roles of health care professionals in various delivery systems.

c. Family and other support systems of the individual.

**10.1 CLINICAL JUDGMENTS AND RELATED SKILLS** needed to refer individuals and their families to appropriate resources when necessary to meet health needs.

a. Identify providers and resources to meet patient/client needs.

b. Assist individuals to communicate needs to their support systems and other health care providers.

**11. KNOWLEDGE NEEDED TO FUNCTION WITHIN THE ORGANIZATIONAL STRUCTURE OF VARIOUS HEALTH CARE SETTINGS.**

a. Principles of organizational behavior.

b. Relationships between nursing, medical, and administrative components of the organization.

c. Types of organizational structures and their interrelationships in health care settings.

d. Individual and group responses to anticipated change in organizations.

e. Individual, organizational, and environmental factors that promote or inhibit change.

f. Strategies for initiating and facilitating change.

g. Methods for containing health care costs.

h. Methods for promoting safety.

**11.1 CLINICAL JUDGMENTS AND RELATED SKILLS** needed to facilitate changes in health care.
   a. Identify activities that, if changed, would improve health care.
   b. Participate in planning, implementing, and evaluating changes that lead to improvement in the work setting.

**11.2 CLINICAL JUDGMENTS AND RELATED SKILLS** needed to promote cost containment through appropriate use of human and material resources.
   a. Select human and material resources that are optimal, legal, and cost effective.
   b. Identify problems and work with other providers to resolve them.

**11.3 CLINICAL JUDGMENTS AND RELATED SKILLS** needed to promote a safe environment for patients/clients and health care providers.
   a. Monitor effectiveness and safety of the environment and equipment.
   b. Refer problems to appropriate individuals.

*MEMBER OF A PROFESSION*

   The nurse as a member of a profession assumes responsibility for the quality of nursing care for patients/clients in his or her immediate case load as well as for others in the clinical setting. The nurse applies knowledge and research findings to practice and raises questions for further research about how practice should be conducted in a changing health care environment. The nurse is aware of legislative, regulatory, ethical, and professional standards that define the scope of practice. As a professional, the nurse aspires to improve the discipline of nursing and its contribution to society through participation in professional organizations and the use of the political process. The professional nurse is committed to the value of collegiality and the need for life-long learning and continual growth toward expert practice.

**12. KNOWLEDGE NEEDED TO DEMONSTRATE ACCOUNTABILITY FOR OWN NURSING PRACTICE.**
   a. Established standards and definitions of nursing practice.
   b. Codes of ethics concerning nurses and nursing practice.
   c. Legal parameters of nursing practice and health care.
   d. Historical and political aspects of nursing as a profession.
   e. Issues and trends affecting the nursing role and health care delivery.
   f. Process of self-evaluation to determine learning needs.

g. Sources of appropriate continuing education.

h. Implications of theoretical and technological changes for nursing practice.

**12.1 PROFESSIONAL JUDGMENTS AND RELATED SKILLS** needed to practice responsibly and accountably within legal, ethical, professional, and institutional parameters.

a. Evaluate own level of practice and seek methods for improvement.

b. Identify mechanisms for resolving concerns and conflicts related to practice.

**12.2 PROFESSIONAL JUDGMENTS AND RELATED SKILLS** needed to recognize own learning needs and seek opportunities to meet them.

a. Establish goals and set a plan for achieving them.

b. Identify and participate in formal and informal educational offerings.

c. Evaluate progress toward achieving one's goals.

**13. KNOWLEDGE NEEDED TO SERVE AS A HEALTH CARE ADVOCATE IN MONITORING AND ENSURING THE QUALITY OF HEALTH CARE PRACTICES.**

a. The role of the health care advocate and the advocacy process.

b. Rights and responsibilities of people relative to health care.

c. Methods for evaluating the quality of nursing practice and health care.

d. Formal and informal sources of power to initiate change.

e. The interactive nature of the sociopolitical, economic, and legislative arenas and the system of health care delivery.

**13.1 PROFESSIONAL JUDGMENTS AND RELATED SKILLS** needed to act as a health care advocate.

a. Identify health needs that are not being met.

b. Promote collaboration with other professional resources and agencies.

**13.2 PROFESSIONAL JUDGMENTS AND RELATED SKILLS** needed to participate in evaluation of nursing practice through quality assurance programs.

a. Compare quality of care and outcomes with established standards.

b. Identify change strategies appropriate to the improvement of care.

c. Evaluate effectiveness of changes in care.

**13.3 PROFESSIONAL JUDGMENTS AND RELATED SKILLS** needed to participate in monitoring nursing and health care services to ensure safe, legal, and ethical health care practices.
   a. Compare observed care to established standards for appropriate care.
   b. Take action to correct health care practices not meeting established standards.

**14. KNOWLEDGE NEEDED TO PROMOTE NURSING AS A PROFESSION.**
   a. Trends and issues confronting nursing and health care.
   b. Methods of organizing groups of people to bring about change.
   c. Existence and functions of major nursing organizations.
   d. Political action process.

**14.1 PROFESSIONAL JUDGMENTS AND RELATED SKILLS** needed to support activities of the profession that improve nursing and health care delivery and advance the discipline of nursing.
   a. Participate in activities that focus on health care improvement.
   b. Promote consumer awareness of nursing's contribution to health promotion and health care delivery.
   c. Promote collegiality and collectivity among nurses.

## CONCLUSIONS

In this document, we have recommended the essential education for the professional nurse. These essentials provide a standard by which faculty can measure the content of the curriculum and the performance of the graduate. When the essentials have been incorporated into nursing curricula, employers of nurses can use them as a base for new graduate orientation programs. The essentials also provide a solid foundation for future personal and professional growth of individual students and graduates as well as for the development of the nursing profession itself.

Program length and the structure and implementation of the curriculum are the responsibility of the faculty of each academic institution, however, college and university students in all nursing programs should obtain the essentials identified for the first professional degree in nursing. Traditionally, the first professional degree in nursing has been the baccalaureate. The Panel believes these essentials can be achieved within a baccalaureate program. We challenge faculty to review and revise, if needed, curricular content and teaching strategies to achieve this goal. **We recommend that the American Association of Colleges of Nursing review and revise this document in three to five years.**

# BIBLIOGRAPHY

Association of American Colleges. 1985. INTEGRITY IN THE COLLEGE CURRICULUM. Washington, DC: Project on Redefining the Meaning and Purpose of Baccalaureate Degrees, American Association of Colleges. (Complete text printed in THE CHRONICLE OF HIGHER EDUCATION, XXIX:22, February 13, 1985.)

American Nurses' Association. 1976. CODE FOR NURSES WITH INTERPRETIVE STATEMENTS. Kansas City, MO: American Nurses' Association.

Institute of Medicine. 1983. NURSING AND NURSING EDUCATION: PUBLIC POLICIES AND PRIVATE ACTIONS. Washington, DC: Committee on Nursing and Nursing Education, Institute of Medicine.

National Commission on Nursing. 1983. SUMMARY REPORT AND RECOMMENDATIONS. Chicago, IL: American Hospital Association.

National Endowment for the Humanities. 1984. TO RECLAIM A LEGACY. Washington, DC: Study Group on the State of Learning in the Humanities in Higher Education, National Endowment for the Humanities. (Complete text printed in THE CHRONICLE OF HIGHER EDUCATION, XXIX:14, November 28, 1984.)

National Institute of Education. 1984. INVOLVEMENT IN LEARNING: REALIZING THE POTENTIAL OF AMERICAN HIGHER EDUCATION. Study Group on the Conditions of Excellence in American Higher Education. Washington, DC: U.S. Department of Education. (Complete text printed in THE CHRONICLE OF HIGHER EDUCATION, XXIX:9, October 24, 1984.)

The Essentials Report was endorsed by the members of the American Association of Colleges of Nursing at the October 1986 Semi-Annual Meeting in Washington, DC. The Board of Directors was instructed to develop plans for implementation of the essentials.

A major publication is being prepared that will include a description of the conduct and results of the Project, background papers commissioned for the Project, and papers defining appropriate teaching and evaluation strategies related to the implementation of the essentials.

# APPENDIX

## NURSING INTERVENTIONS AND CLINICAL SKILLS

All skills, regardless of the level of achievement, will be performed safely, focus on acceptable outcomes, and cause no undue physical or psychosocial harm. The term *supervision* denotes the need for validation of skill performance, rather than the need for instruction. Three levels of achievement are used to describe the practice of the entry level professional nurse.

### Key for Achievement Levels

PROFICIENT:    Able to make clinical judgments and carry out related nursing interventions without supervision and adapt them to patients/clients in a variety of situations.

INTERMEDIATE: Able to make clinical judgments and carry out related nursing interventions with limited supervision.

BEGINNING:    Able to make clinical judgments and carry out related nursing intervention with supervision.

Clinical judgments and nursing interventions at the proficient level have been carried out in multiple clinical settings and those at the intermediate level in at least one setting. Clinical judgments and interventions at the beginning level have been practiced in a laboratory setting and, in some instances, in a clinical setting.

In the determination of the minimal level of achievement for the essentials, the panel and work groups took a number of considerations in mind including relationship to clinical judgment, availability of clinical experiences, complexity, and importance to professional practice.

**The panel recommends that graduates of all professional nursing programs possess the nursing interventions and clinical skills necessary to make clinical judgments.** The following table presents examples of nursing interventions and clinical skills with designated achievement levels for three roles of the nurse: provider of care, coordinator of care, and member of a profession. The provider of care section is furthered organized by assessment, intervention, and evaluation skills. Some graduates will exceed the designated level of achievement initially; many will do so after an orientation. Graduates are expected to proceed to higher levels of achievement on an individual basis.

## EXAMPLES OF NURSING INTERVENTIONS AND CLINICAL SKILLS AND LEVEL OF ACHIEVEMENT

*PROVIDER OF CARE*
  *Assessment Skills* such as:
    Proficient:  Measure height and weight
                 Measure vital signs
                 Obtain body measurements
                 Obtain clean urinary specimen
                 Use communication skills

*Assessment Skills* (cont.)
Intermediate: Assess health status using interview, inspection, palpation, percussion, and auscultation
Determine priorities
Insert intravenous needle
Insert urinary catheter
Obtain culture and blood specimen
Set goals
Solve assessment problems
Use collaboration, coordination, and observation skills

Beginning: Administer developmental, functional, and psychosocial screening tools
Use consultation skills

*Intervention Skills* such as:
Proficient: Administer enema
Administer oral, topical, sub-cutaneous and intramuscular medications
Administer oxygen
Administer Sitz bath
Apply anti-embolic hose
Apply hot and cold packs
Apply siderails
Apply soft restraints
Assist to ambulate with walker, cane, and crutches
Assist to change environment
Assist to cough and deep breathe
Calculate medication dosage
Conduct change of shift report
Feed by mouth
Make occupied, unoccupied, and surgical beds
Manage intravenous therapy
Manage naso-gastric tube
Manage urinary catheter
Measure intake and output
Monitor medication effects and side effects
Monitor nutritional intake- calories, nutrients, fluids, and electrolytes
Promote physical exercise
Provide hair and nail care and oral hygiene
Provide range of motion exercises
Provide skin care- give back rub and monitor for breakdown
Record health data
Suction nose and throat
Transfer to chair, wheelchair, and stretcher
Transport in wheelchair and stretcher
Use basic and surgical handwashing techniques
Use communication skills
Use positioning skills
Use sterile technique

Intermediate: Adapt diet to preferences and needs
Administer basic cardiac life support (BCLS Certified)
Administer cast care
Administer Heimlich maneuver

Administer intravenous medication
Administer ostomy care
Assist with vaginal examination
Attach piggy-back fluid
Change dressing
Conduct patient/client interview
Determine priorities
Encourage relaxation techniques
Establish airway
Evaluate clinical data and research findings
Facilitate group process
Feed by gastrostomy
Insert intravenous needle
Insert naso-gastric tube
Insert urinary catheter
Irrigate urinary catheter
Locate emergency equipment and drugs
Maintain heparin lock
Maintain isolation technique
Make decisions
Modify environment to increase sensory stimulation
Monitor response to ventilator
Provide anticipatory guidance
Provide bladder and bowel training
Provide health teaching
Provide pulmonary hygiene
Record emergency team activities
Retrieve information
Search literature
Solve intervention problems
Use collaboration, coordination, negotiation, observation, and organizational skills
Use teaching skills- contracting and discussion
Use therapeutic communication- attending, clarifying, coaching, counseling, facilitating, and touching

Beginning: Administer intravenous push, blood, and blood products
Apply splint
Apply traction apparatus
Assist with biopsy
Assist with spinal tap
Control hemorrhage
Insert airway
Manage chest tube and surgical drain
Monitor psychological crisis
Provide basic first aid
Provide tracheotomy care
Use change strategies
Use computer for information storing and retrieval
Use crisis interventions skills
Use teaching skills- demonstration and role playing

*Evaluation Skills*, such as:
     Proficient:   Record health data
                     Use communication skills

     Intermediate:   Administer evaluation tools
                     Collaborate with colleagues
                     Determine criteria
                     Determine priorities
                     Measure health outcomes
                     Revise goals
                     Solve evaluation problems
                     Use observation skills

     Beginning:   Analyze results of evaluation tool

## COORDINATOR OF CARE
*Clinical skills* such as
     Proficient:   Record health data
                     Use communication skills

     Intermediate:   Assist individual and family to use community resources
                     Demonstrate an assertive manner
                     Facilitate group process
                     Measure health outcomes
                     Solve coordination problems
                     Use collaboration, coordination, delegation, leadership, negotiation, and organizational skills
                     Use observation skills
                     Use referral techniques
                     Use teaching skills
                     Use therapeutic communication: coaching and counseling

     Beginning:   Resolve conflict
                     Use change strategies

## MEMBER OF A PROFESSION
*Professional skills*, such as
     Proficient:   Use communication skills

     Intermediate:   Determine priorities
                     Facilitate group process
                     Set goals
                     Solve problems
                     Use an assertive manner
                     Use collaboration, leadership, and negotiation skills
                     Use observation skills

     Beginning:   Use change strategies

# Appendix B:

## Summary of American Baccalaureate and Graduate Nursing Education Programs

| Institution and State | City | GN | RN | MS | DC | PD* |
|---|---|---|---|---|---|---|
| **ALABAMA** | | | | | | |
| Auburn Univ. | Auburn University | X | X | | | |
| Auburn Univ. at Montgomery | Montgomery | X | X | | | |
| Jacksonville State Univ. | Jacksonville | X | | | | |
| Oakwood College | Huntsville | | X | | | |
| Samford Univ. | Birmingham | X | X | | | |
| The Univ. of Alabama | Tuscaloosa | X | X | | | |
| Troy State Univ. | Troy | X | X | X | | |
| Tuskegee Univ. | Tuskegee | X | X | | | |
| Univ. of Alabama at Birmingham | Birmingham | X | X | X | X | X |
| Univ. of Alabama-Huntsville | Huntsville | X | X | X | | |
| Univ. of North Alabama | Florence | X | X | | | |
| Univ. of South Alabama | Mobile | X | X | X | | |

(continued)

| Institution and State | City | GN | RN | MS | DC | PD* |
|---|---|---|---|---|---|---|
| **ALASKA** | | | | | | |
| Univ. of Alaska Anchorage | Anchorage | X | X | X | | |
| **ARIZONA** | | | | | | |
| Arizona State Univ. | Tempe | X | X | X | | |
| Grand Canyon Univ. | Phoenix | X | X | | | |
| Northern Arizona Univ. | Flagstaff | X | X | | | |
| Univ. of Arizona | Tucson | X | X | X | X | X |
| Univ. of Phoenix | Phoenix | | X | X | | |
| **ARKANSAS** | | | | | | |
| Arkansas State Univ. | State University | X | X | | | |
| Arkansas Tech Univ. | Russellville | X | X | | | |
| Harding Univ. | Searcy | X | X | | | |
| Henderson State Univ. | Arkadelphia | X | X | | | |
| Univ. of Arkansas at Pine Bluff | Pine Bluff | X | X | | | |
| Univ. of Arkansas for Med. Sciences | Little Rock | X | X | X | | |
| Univ. of Arkansas-Monticello | Monticello | | X | | | |
| Univ. of Central Arkansas | Conway | X | X | X | | |
| **CALIFORNIA** | | | | | | |
| Azusa Pacific Univ. | Azusa | X | X | X | | |
| California State Univ.-Bakersfield | Bakersfield | X | X | X | | |
| California State Univ.-Chico | Chico | X | | X | | |
| California State Univ.-Fresno | Fresno | X | X | X | | |

*(continued)*

---

*Key to Programs Offered: GN = Generic Baccalaureate; RN = RN Baccalaureate; MS = Master's; DC = Doctoral; PD = Postdoctoral*

192

| Institution and State | City | GN | RN | MS | DC | PD* |
|---|---|---|---|---|---|---|
| California State Univ.-Fullerton | Fullerton | | X | | | |
| California State Univ.-Long Beach | Long Beach | X | X | X | | |
| California State Univ.-Los Angeles | Los Angeles | X | X | X | | |
| California State Univ.-Sacramento | Sacramento | X | | X | | |
| Cal. State Univ.-San Bernardino | San Bernardino | | X | | | |
| California State Univ.-Stanislaus | Turlock | | X | | | |
| Dominican College of San Rafael | San Rafael | X | X | | | |
| Holy Names College | Oakland | | X | | | |
| Humboldt State Univ. | Arcata | X | X | | | |
| Loma Linda Univ. | Loma Linda | X | X | X | | |
| Mt. St. Mary's College | Los Angeles | X | X | | | |
| Samuel Merritt-Saint Mary's | Oakland | X | X | | | |
| San Diego State Univ. | San Diego | X | | X | | |
| San Francisco State Univ. | San Francisco | X | X | X | | |
| San Jose State Univ. | San Jose | X | | X | | |
| Sonoma State Univ. | Rohnert Park | | X | X | | |
| Univ. of California-Los Angeles | Los Angeles | X | X | X | X | |
| Univ. of California-San Francisco | San Francisco | | | X | X | |
| Univ. of San Diego | San Diego | | X | X | X | |
| Univ. of San Francisco | San Francisco | X | X | X | | |
| Univ. of Southern California | Los Angeles | X | X | X | | |

(continued)

| Institution and State | City | GN | RN | MS | DC | PD* |
|---|---|:---:|:---:|:---:|:---:|:---:|
| **COLORADO** | | | | | | |
| Mesa State College | Grand Junction | X | X | | | |
| Metropolitan State College | Denver | | X | | | |
| Univ. of Colorado Health Sci. Ctr. | Denver | X | X | X | X | |
| Univ. of Northern Colorado | Greeley | X | | X | | |
| **CONNECTICUT** | | | | | | |
| Fairfield Univ. | Fairfield | X | X | | | |
| Sacred Heart Univ. | Fairfield | X | X | | | |
| Southern Connecticut State Univ. | New Haven | X | X | X | | |
| St. Joseph College | West Hartford | X | X | X | | |
| Univ. of Bridgeport | Bridgeport | X | X | | | |
| Univ. of Connecticut | Storrs | X | X | X | | |
| Univ. of Hartford | West Hartford | | X | X | | |
| Western Connecticut State Univ. | Danbury | X | X | X | | |
| Yale Univ. | New Haven | | | X | | |
| **DELAWARE** | | | | | | |
| Delaware State College | Dover | X | X | | | |
| Univ. of Delaware | Newark | X | X | X | | |
| Wesley College | Dover | | X | | | |
| Wilmington College | New Castle | | X | | | |
| **DISTRICT OF COLUMBIA** | | | | | | |
| Catholic Univ. of America | Washington | X | X | X | X | |
| Georgetown Univ. | Washington | X | X | X | | |
| Howard Univ. | Washington | X | X | X | | |

*(continued)*

---

*Key to Programs Offered: **GN** = Generic Baccalaureate; **RN** = RN Baccalaureate; **MS** = Master's; **DC** = Doctoral; **PD** = Postdoctoral

| Institution and State | City | GN | RN | MS | DC | PD* |
|---|---|---|---|---|---|---|
| **FLORIDA** | | | | | | |
| Barry Univ. | Miami Shores | X | X | X | | |
| Bethune-Cookman College | Daytona Beach | X | X | | | |
| Florida Atlantic Univ. | Boca Raton | X | X | X | | |
| Florida International Univ. | North Miami | X | X | | | |
| Florida Southern College | Lakeland | | X | | | |
| Florida State Univ. | Tallahassee | X | X | X | | |
| Jacksonville Univ. | Jacksonville | X | | | | |
| Pensacola Christian College | Pensacola | X | X | | | |
| Univ. of Central Florida | Orlando | X | X | | | |
| Univ. of Florida | Gainesville | X | X | X | X | |
| Univ. of Miami | Miami | X | X | X | X | |
| Univ. of North Florida | Jacksonville | X | X | | | |
| Univ. of South Florida | Tampa | X | X | X | | |
| Univ. of Tampa | Tampa | | X | | | |
| Univ. of West Florida | Pensacola | | X | | | |
| **GEORGIA** | | | | | | |
| Albany State College | Albany | X | X | X | | |
| Armstrong State College | Savannah | X | X | X | | |
| Brenau College | Gainesville | X | X | | | |
| Clayton State College | Morrow | | X | | | |
| Emory Univ. | Atlanta | X | X | X | | |
| Georgia College | Milledgeville | X | X | X | | |
| Georgia Southern College | Statesboro | X | X | X | | |

(continued)

| Institution and State | City | GN | RN | MS | DC | PD* |
|---|---|---|---|---|---|---|
| Georgia Southwestern College | Americus | | X | | | |
| Georgia State Univ. | Atlanta | X | X | X | X | |
| Kennesaw College | Marietta | X | | | | |
| Medical College of Georgia | Augusta | X | X | X | X | X |
| North Georgia College | Dahlonega | | X | | | |
| Valdosta State College | Valdosta | X | X | X | | |

**GUAM**

| | | | | | | |
|---|---|---|---|---|---|---|
| Univ. of Guam | Mangilao | X | X | | | |

**HAWAII**

| | | | | | | |
|---|---|---|---|---|---|---|
| Hawaii Loa College | Kaneohe | X | X | | | |
| Univ. of Hawaii at Manoa | Honolulu | X | X | X | | |

**IDAHO**

| | | | | | | |
|---|---|---|---|---|---|---|
| Boise State Univ. | Boise | X | X | | | |
| Idaho State Univ. | Pocatello | X | | X | | |
| Lewis Clark State College | Lewiston | | X | | | |

**ILLINOIS**

| | | | | | | |
|---|---|---|---|---|---|---|
| Aurora Univ. | Aurora | X | X | X | | |
| Barat College & Univ. of Hlth. Sci. | North Chicago | | X | | | |
| Bradley Univ. | Peoria | X | X | X | | |
| Chicago State Univ. | Chicago | X | X | | | |
| Concordia-W. Suburban Col. of Nursing | Oak Park | X | X | | | |
| DePaul Univ. | Chicago | X | X | X | | |
| Elmhurst College | Elmhurst | X | X | | | |

(continued)

*Key to Programs Offered:  GN = Generic Baccalaureate; RN = RN Baccalaureate; MS = Master's; DC = Doctoral; PD = Postdoctoral

| Institution and State | City | GN | RN | MS | DC | PD* |
|---|---|---|---|---|---|---|
| Governors State Univ. | Univ. Park | | X | X | | |
| Illinois Benedictine College | Lisle | | X | | | |
| Illinois Wesleyan Univ. | Bloomington | X | X | | | |
| Lewis Univ. | Romeoville | X | X | X | | |
| Loyola Univ. of Chicago | Chicago | X | | X | X | |
| MacMurray College | Jacksonville | X | X | | | |
| McKendree College | Lebanon | | X | | | |
| Millikin Univ. | Decatur | X | X | | | |
| North Park College | Chicago | X | X | | | |
| Northern Illinois Univ. | DeKalb | X | X | X | | |
| Northwestern Univ. | Chicago | X | X | X | | |
| Olivet Nazarene Univ. | Kankakee | X | X | | | |
| Quincy College | Quincy | X | X | | | |
| Rockford College | Rockford | X | X | | | |
| Rush Univ. | Chicago | X | X | X | X | X |
| Sangamon State Univ. | Springfield | | X | | | |
| St. Xavier College | Chicago | X | X | X | | |
| Trinity Christian College | Palos Heights | X | X | | | |
| Univ. of Illinois | Chicago | X | X | X | X | |

## INDIANA

| Institution and State | City | GN | RN | MS | DC | PD* |
|---|---|---|---|---|---|---|
| Anderson Univ. | Anderson | X | X | | | |
| Ball State Univ. | Muncie | X | X | X | | |
| Bethel College of Indiana | Mishawaka | X | X | | | |
| DePauw Univ. | Greencastle | X | | | | |
| Goshen College | Goshen | X | X | | | |
| Indiana State Univ. | Terre Haute | X | | X | | |
| Indiana Univ. | Indianapolis | X | X | X | X | |

(continued)

| Institution and State | City | GN | RN | MS | DC | PD* |
|---|---|:-:|:-:|:-:|:-:|:-:|
| Indiana Univ.-Purdue Univ. | Fort Wayne | | X | | | |
| Indiana Wesleyan Univ. | Marion | X | X | X | | |
| Purdue Univ.-Calumet Campus | Hammond | | X | X | | |
| Purdue Univ. | West Lafayette | X | | | | |
| Saint Francis College | Fort Wayne | X | | | | |
| Saint Mary's College | Notre Dame | X | | | | |
| The Univ. of Indianapolis | Indianapolis | X | X | | | |
| Univ. of Evansville | Evansville | X | X | X | | |
| Univ. of Southern Indiana | Evansville | X | X | | | |
| Valparaiso Univ. | Valparaiso | X | X | X | | |

## IOWA

| Institution and State | City | GN | RN | MS | DC | PD* |
|---|---|:-:|:-:|:-:|:-:|:-:|
| Briar Cliff College | Sioux City | X | X | | | |
| Buena Vista College | Fort Dodge | | X | | | |
| Clarke College | Dubuque | X | X | | | |
| Coe College | Cedar Rapids | X | X | | | |
| Drake Univ. | Des Moines | | X | X | | |
| Grand View College | Des Moines | X | X | | | |
| Luther College | Decorah | X | X | | | |
| Morningside College | Sioux City | X | X | | | |
| Mount Mercy College | Cedar Rapids | X | X | | | |
| Univ. of Dubuque | Dubuque | | X | X | | |
| Univ. of Iowa | Iowa City | X | X | X | X | |

## KANSAS

| Institution and State | City | GN | RN | MS | DC | PD* |
|---|---|:-:|:-:|:-:|:-:|:-:|
| Bethel College of Kansas | North Newton | X | X | | | |
| Fort Hays State Univ. | Hays | X | X | X | | |

(continued)

*Key to Programs Offered: GN = Generic Baccalaureate; RN = RN Baccalaureate; MS = Master's; DC = Doctoral; PD = Postdoctoral

198

| Institution and State | City | GN | RN | MS | DC | PD* |
|---|---|---|---|---|---|---|
| Kansas Newman College | Wichita | | X | | | |
| Kansas Wesleyan Univ. | Salina | | X | | | |
| Mid-America Nazarene College | Olathe | X | X | | | |
| Pittsburg State Univ. | Pittsburg | X | X | | | |
| Southwestern College | Winfield | X | X | | | |
| St. Mary College | Leavenworth | | X | | | |
| St. Mary of the Plains College | Wichita | X | X | | | |
| The Wichita State Univ. | Wichita | X | X | X | | |
| Univ. of Kansas Medical Center | Kansas City | X | X | X | X | |
| Washburn Univ. of Topeka | Topeka | X | X | | | |
| **KENTUCKY** | | | | | | |
| Berea College | Berea | X | | | | |
| Kentucky Wesleyan College | Owensboro | | X | | | |
| Morehead State Univ. | Morehead | X | X | | | |
| Northern Kentucky Univ. | Highland Heights | | X | | | |
| Spalding Univ. | Louisville | X | X | X | | |
| Thomas More College | Crestview Hills | X | X | | | |
| Univ. of Kentucky | Lexington | X | X | X | X | |
| Univ. of Louisville | Louisville | X | X | X | | |
| Western Kentucky Univ. | Bowling Green | X | X | | | |

(continued)

| Institution and State | City | GN | RN | MS | DC | PD* |
|---|---|---|---|---|---|---|
| **LOUISIANA** | | | | | | |
| Louisiana College | Pineville | X | X | | | |
| Louisiana State Univ. Medical Ctr. | New Orleans | X | | | X | X |
| Loyola Univ. of New Orleans | New Orleans | | X | | | |
| McNeese State Univ. | Lake Charles | X | X | X | | |
| Northeast Louisiana Univ. | Monroe | X | X | | | |
| Our Lady of Holy Cross College | New Orleans | X | | | | |
| Southeastern Louisiana Univ. | Hammond | X | X | X | | |
| Southern Univ. and A&M College | Baton Rouge | X | | | | |
| Univ. of Southwestern Louisiana | Lafayette | X | | | | |
| **MAINE** | | | | | | |
| Husson College/E. Maine Medical Ctr | Bangor | X | X | | | |
| St. Joseph's College | Windham | X | X | | | |
| Univ. of Maine | Orono | X | X | | | |
| Univ. of Maine-Fort Kent | Fort Kent | X | X | | | |
| Univ. of Southern Maine | Portland | X | X | X | | |
| **MARYLAND** | | | | | | |
| College of Notre Dame of Maryland | Baltimore | | X | | | |
| Columbia Union College | Takoma Park | X | X | | | |
| Coppin State College | Baltimore | X | X | | | |

*(continued)*

---

*Key to Programs Offered: **GN** = Generic Baccalaureate; **RN** = RN Baccalaureate; **MS** = Master's; **DC** = Doctoral; **PD** = Postdoctoral

| Institution and State | City | GN | RN | MS | DC | PD* |
|---|---|---|---|---|---|---|
| Johns Hopkins Univ. | Baltimore | X | | X | X | |
| Salisbury State Univ. | Salisbury | X | X | X | | |
| Towson State Univ. | Towson | X | X | | | |
| Univ. of Maryland-Baltimore | Baltimore | X | X | X | X | |

## MASSACHUSETTS

| | | | | | | |
|---|---|---|---|---|---|---|
| American International College | Springfield | X | X | | | |
| Anna Maria College | Paxton | | X | X | | |
| Assumption College | Gardner | | X | | | |
| Atlantic Union College | South Lancaster | | X | | | |
| Boston College | Chestnut Hill | X | | X | X | |
| College of Our Lady of the Elms | Chicopee | X | | | | |
| Curry College | Milton | X | | | | |
| Emanuel College | Boston | | X | | | |
| Fitchburg State College | Fitchburg | X | X | | | |
| Framingham State College | Framingham | | X | | | |
| Massachusetts College of Pharmacy/Allied Health Sciences | Boston | | X | | | |
| MGH Institute of Health Professions | Boston | | | X | | |
| Northeastern Univ. | Boston | X | X | X | | |
| Regis College | Weston | | X | | | |
| Salem State College | Salem | X | X | X | | |
| Southeastern Massachusetts Univ. | North Dartmouth | X | X | X | | |
| Univ. of Massachusetts-Amherst | Amherst | X | X | X | | |

(continued)

| Institution and State | City | GN | RN | MS | DC | PD* |
|---|---|---|---|---|---|---|
| Univ. of Massachusetts-Boston | Boston | X | | X | | |
| Univ. of Massachusetts Medical Ctr. | Worcester | | | X | | |
| Univ. of Lowell | Lowell | X | X | X | | |
| **MICHIGAN** | | | | | | |
| Eastern Michigan Univ. | Ypsilanti | X | X | | | |
| Ferris State Univ. | Big Rapids | | X | | | |
| Grand Valley State Univ. | Allendale | X | X | X | | |
| Hope/Calvin Colleges | Holland | X | | | | |
| Lake Superior State Univ. | Sault St. Marie | X | X | | | |
| Madonna College | Livonia | X | X | X | | |
| Mercy College of Detroit | Detroit | X | X | | | |
| Michigan State Univ. | East Lansing | X | X | X | | |
| Nazareth College in Kalamazoo | Kalamazoo | X | X | | | |
| Northern Michigan Univ. | Marquette | X | X | X | | |
| Oakland Univ. | Rochester | X | X | X | | |
| Saginaw Valley State Univ. | Univ. Center | X | | X | | |
| Univ. of Michigan, UMMC | Ann Arbor | X | X | X | X | X |
| Wayne State Univ. | Detroit | X | X | X | X | |
| **MINNESOTA** | | | | | | |
| Augsburg College | Minneapolis | | X | | | |
| Bemidji State Univ. | Bemedji | | X | | | |

*(continued)*

---

**\*Key to Programs Offered:** **GN** = Generic Baccalaureate; **RN** = RN Baccalaureate; **MS** = Master's; **DC** = Doctoral; **PD** = Postdoctoral

| Institution and State | City | GN | RN | MS | DC | PD* |
|---|---|---|---|---|---|---|
| Bethel College of Minnesota | St. Paul | X | X | | | |
| College of St. Benedict | St. Joseph | X | X | | | |
| College of St. Scholastica | Duluth | X | | X | | |
| Metropolitan State Univ. | St. Paul | | X | | | |
| Minnesota Intercollegiate Nursing | St. Paul | X | X | | | |
| Moorhead State Univ. | Moorhead | | X | | | |
| Univ. of Minnesota | Minneapolis | X | X | X | X | |
| Winona State Univ. | Winona | X | X | X | | |

**MISSISSIPPI**

| Institution and State | City | GN | RN | MS | DC | PD* |
|---|---|---|---|---|---|---|
| Alcorn State Univ. | Natchez | X | X | | | |
| Delta State Univ. | Cleveland | X | X | | | |
| Mississippi College | Clinton | X | X | | | |
| Mississippi Univ. for Women | Columbus | X | X | X | | |
| Univ. of Mississippi | Jackson | X | X | X | | |
| Univ. of Southern Mississippi | Hattiesburg | X | X | X | | |

**MISSOURI**

| Institution and State | City | GN | RN | MS | DC | PD* |
|---|---|---|---|---|---|---|
| Avila College | Kansas City | X | X | | | |
| Central Methodist College | Fayette | | X | | | |
| Central Missouri State Univ. | Warrensburg | X | X | | | |
| Drury College | Springfield | | X | | | |
| Graceland College | Independence | X | X | | | |
| Maryville College | St. Louis | X | X | | | |
| Missouri Southern State College | Joplin | | X | | | |
| Missouri Western State College | St. Joseph | X | X | | | |

*(continued)*

| Institution and State | City | GN | RN | MS | DC | PD* |
|---|---|---|---|---|---|---|
| Northeast Missouri State Univ. | Kirksville | X | X | | | |
| Research Medical Center | Kansas City | X | X | | | |
| Saint Louis Univ. | Saint Louis | X | X | X | | |
| Southeast Missouri State Univ. | Cape Girardeau | X | X | | | |
| Southwest Baptist Univ. | Springfield | | X | | | |
| Southwest Missouri State Univ. | Springfield | | X | | | |
| Univ. of Missouri-Columbia | Columbia | X | X | X | | |
| Univ. of Missouri-Kansas City | Kansas City | | X | X | | |
| Univ. of Missouri-St. Louis | St. Louis | | X | | | |
| Webster University | Saint Louis | | X | | | |
| William Jewell College | Liberty | X | X | | | |
| **MONTANA** | | | | | | |
| Carroll College | Helena | X | | | | |
| Montana State Univ. | Bozeman | X | X | X | | |
| Northern Montana College | Havre | | X | | | |
| **NEBRASKA** | | | | | | |
| College of Saint Mary | Omaha | | X | | | |
| Creighton Univ. | Omaha | X | X | X | | |
| Kearney State College | Kearney | X | X | | | |
| Midland Lutheran College | Fremont | X | X | | | |

(continued)

*Key to Programs Offered: GN = Generic Baccalaureate; RN = RN Baccalaureate; MS = Master's; DC = Doctoral; PD = Postdoctoral

204

| Institution and State | City | GN | RN | MS | DC | PD* |
|---|---|---|---|---|---|---|
| Nebraska Wesleyan Univ. | Lincoln | | X | | | |
| Union College | Lincoln | X | | | | |
| Univ. of Nebraska | Omaha | X | | X | | |
| **NEVADA** | | | | | | |
| Univ. of Nevada-Las Vegas | Las Vegas | X | X | X | | |
| Univ. of Nevada-Reno | Reno | X | X | X | | |
| **NEW HAMPSHIRE** | | | | | | |
| Saint Anselm College | Manchester | X | X | | | |
| Univ. of New Hampshire | Durham | X | X | X | | |
| **NEW JERSEY** | | | | | | |
| College of St. Elizabeth | Convent Station | | X | | | |
| Fairleigh Dickinson Univ. | Rutherford | X | X | | | |
| Felician College | Lodi | | X | | | |
| Jersey City State College | Jersey City | | X | | | |
| Kean College of New Jersey | Union | | X | | | |
| Monmouth College | West Long Branch | | X | | | |
| Rutgers, The State Univ. of NJ | Newark | X | | | X | X |
| Rutgers, The State Univ.-Camden | Camden | X | X | | | |
| Saint Peter's College | Jersey City | | X | | | |
| Seton Hall Univ. | South Orange | X | X | X | | |
| Stockton State College | Pomona | | X | | | |
| Thomas A. Edison State College | Trenton | | X | | | |

*(continued)*

| Institution and State | City | GN | RN | MS | DC | PD* |
|---|---|---|---|---|---|---|
| Trenton State College | Trenton | X | X | | | |
| William Paterson College | Wayne | X | | | | |
| **NEW MEXICO** | | | | | | |
| New Mexico State Univ. | Las Cruces | | X | | | |
| Univ. of New Mexico | Albuquerque | X | X | X | | |
| **NEW YORK** | | | | | | |
| Adelphi Univ. | Garden City | X | X | X | X | |
| Alfred Univ. | Alfred | X | X | X | | |
| City College of CUNY | New York | X | X | | | |
| College of Mount Saint Vincent | Riverdale | X | X | X | | |
| College of New Rochelle | New Rochelle | X | X | X | | |
| Columbia Univ. Teachers College | New York | | | X | X | |
| Columbia Univ. | New York | X | X | X | | |
| D'Youville College | Buffalo | X | X | X | | |
| Daemen College | Amherst | | X | | | |
| Dominican College of Blauvelt | Orangeburg | X | X | | | |
| Elmira College | Elmira | X | X | | | |
| Hartwick College | Oneonta | X | X | | | |
| Hunter College of CUNY | New York | X | X | X | | |
| Keuka College | Keuka Park | X | X | | | |
| Lehman College of CUNY | Bronx | X | X | X | | |
| Long Island Univ.-Brooklyn | Brooklyn | X | | | | |

*Key to Programs Offered: **GN** = Generic Baccalaureate; **RN** = RN Baccalaureate; **MS** = Master's; **DC** = Doctoral; **PD** = Postdoctoral

| Institution and State | City | GN | RN | MS | DC | PD* |
|---|---|---|---|---|---|---|
| Medgar Evers College of CUNY | Brooklyn | | X | | | |
| Molloy College | Rockville Centre | X | X | X | | |
| Mt. Saint Mary College | Newburgh | X | X | | | |
| Nazareth College of Rochester | Rochester | | X | | | |
| New York Univ. | New York | X | X | X | X | |
| Niagara Univ. | Niagara University | | X | | | |
| Pace Univ. | Pleasantville | X | X | X | | |
| Roberts Wesleyan College | Rochester | X | X | | | |
| Russell Sage College | Troy | X | X | X | | |
| SUNY College at Brockport | Brockport | X | X | | | |
| SUNY College at Plattsburgh | Plattsburgh | X | X | | | |
| SUNY Health Sci. Ctr./Brooklyn | Brooklyn | X | X | X | | |
| SUNY Health Sci. Ctr./Syracuse | Syracuse | | X | X | | |
| SUNY Inst. of Tech. at Utica/Rome | Utica | | X | X | | |
| SUNY/Binghamton | Binghamton | X | X | X | | |
| SUNY/Buffalo | Buffalo | X | X | X | X | |
| SUNY/College at New Paltz | New Paltz | | X | | | |
| SUNY/Stony Brook | Stony Brook | X | X | X | | |
| Syracuse Univ. | Syracuse | X | X | X | | |
| Univ. of the State of New York | Albany | X | X | | | |
| Univ. of Rochester | Rochester | X | X | X | X | X |
| Utica College of Syracuse Univ. | Utica | X | X | | | |
| York College of CUNY | Jamaica Queens | | X | | | |

*(continued)*

| Institution and State | City | GN | RN | MS | DC | PD* |
|---|---|---|---|---|---|---|
| **NORTH CAROLINA** | | | | | | |
| Duke Univ. | Durham | | | X | | |
| East Carolina Univ. | Greenville | X | X | X | | |
| Gardner-Webb College | Boiling Springs | | X | | | |
| Lenoir-Rhyne College | Hickory | X | X | | | |
| North Carolina A&T State Univ. | Greensboro | X | X | | | |
| North Carolina Central Univ. | Durham | X | | | | |
| Queens College | Charlotte | X | | X | | |
| Univ. of North Carolina-Chapel Hill | Chapel Hill | X | X | X | X | |
| Univ. of North Carolina-Charlotte | Charlotte | X | X | X | | |
| Univ. of North Carolina-Greensboro | Greensboro | X | X | X | | |
| Univ. of North Carolina-Wilmington | Wilmington | X | X | | | |
| Western Carolina Univ. | Cullowhee | X | X | | | |
| Winston-Salem State Univ. | Winston-Salem | X | | | | |
| **NORTH DAKOTA** | | | | | | |
| Jamestown College | Jamestown | X | X | | | |
| Minot State College | Minot | X | X | | | |
| Tri-College Univ. | Fargo | X | | | | |
| Univ. of North Dakota | Grand Forks | X | X | X | | |
| **OHIO** | | | | | | |
| Ashland Univ. | Ashland | | X | | | |
| Bluffton College | Bluffton | | X | | | |

*(continued)*

---

**\*Key to Programs Offered:** **GN** = Generic Baccalaureate; **RN** = RN Baccalaureate; **MS** = Master's; **DC** = Doctoral; **PD** = Postdoctoral

208

| Institution and State | City | GN | RN | MS | DC | PD* |
|---|---|---|---|---|---|---|
| Capital Univ. | Columbus | X | X | | | |
| Case Western Reserve Univ. | Cleveland | | | X | X | |
| Cedarville College | Cedarville | X | X | | | |
| Cleveland State Univ. | Cleveland | X | X | | | |
| College of Mount St. Joseph | Mount St. Joseph | X | X | | | |
| Franklin Univ. | Columbus | | X | | | |
| Lourdes College | Sylvania | | X | | | |
| Medical College of Ohio | Toledo | X | X | X | | |
| Ohio State Univ. | Columbus | X | X | X | X | |
| Ohio Univ. | Athens | | X | | | |
| Ohio Wesleyan Univ. | Delaware | X | | | | |
| Univ. of Akron | Akron | X | X | X | | |
| Univ. of Cincinnati | Cincinnati | X | X | X | | |
| Ursuline College | Pepper Pike | X | | | | |
| Walsh College | Canton | | X | | | |
| Wright State Univ. | Dayton | X | X | X | | |
| Xavier Univ. | Cincinnati | | X | | | |
| Youngstown State Univ. | Youngstown | X | | | | |
| **OKLAHOMA** | | | | | | |
| Central State Univ. | Edmond | X | X | | | |
| East Central Univ. | Ada | X | X | | | |
| Langston Univ. | Langston | X | X | | | |
| Northeastern State Univ. | Tahlequah | | X | | | |
| Northwestern Oklahoma State Univ. | Alva | X | X | | | |
| Oklahoma City Univ. | Oklahoma City | X | X | | | |
| Oral Roberts Univ. | Tulsa | X | | X | | |

(continued)

| Institution and State | City | GN | RN | MS | DC | PD* |
|---|---|---|---|---|---|---|
| Southern Nazarene Univ. | Bethany | X | X | | | |
| Southwestern Oklahoma State Univ. | Weatherford | X | X | | | |
| The Univ. of Tulsa | Tulsa | X | X | | | |
| Univ. of Oklahoma | Oklahoma City | X | X | X | | |
| **OREGON** | | | | | | |
| Linfield College | Portland | X | X | | | |
| Oregon Health Sciences Univ. | Portland | X | X | X | X | X |
| Oregon Institute of Technology | Klamath Falls | X | X | | | |
| Univ. of Portland | Portland | X | | X | | |
| Walla Walla College | Portland | X | | | | |
| **PENNSYLVANIA** | | | | | | |
| Albright College | Reading | X | X | | | |
| Allentown College | Center Valley | X | X | X | | |
| Bloomsburg Univ. | Bloomsburg | X | X | X | | |
| California Univ. of Pennsylvania | California | | | X | | |
| Carlow College | Pittsburgh | X | X | | | |
| Cedar Crest College | Allentown | X | X | | | |
| Duquesne Univ. | Pittsburgh | X | X | X | | |
| East Stroudsburg Univ. | East Stroudsburg | X | X | | | |
| Eastern College | St. Davids | | X | | | |
| Edinboro Univ. of Pennsylvania | Edinboro | X | X | X | | |
| Gannon Univ. | Erie | X | X | X | | |
| Gwynedd-Mercy College | Gwynedd Valley | | X | X | | |
| Hahnemann Univ. | Philadelphia | | X | | | |
| Holy Family College | Philadelphia | X | X | | | |

*(continued)*

---

*Key to Programs Offered: **GN** = Generic Baccalaureate; **RN** = RN Baccalaureate; **MS** = Master's; **DC** = Doctoral; **PD** = Postdoctoral

| Institution and State | City | GN | RN | MS | DC | PD* |
|---|---|---|---|---|---|---|
| Immaculata College | Immaculata | | X | | | |
| Indiana Univ. of Pennsylvania | Indiana | X | X | X | | |
| Kutztown Univ. | Kutztown | X | | | | |
| La Roche College | Pittsburgh | | X | X | | |
| La Salle Univ. | Philadelphia | | X | X | | |
| Lycoming College | Williamsport | X | X | | | |
| Mansfield Univ. | Mansfield | X | | | | |
| Marywood College | Scranton | X | X | | | |
| Messiah College | Grantham | X | X | | | |
| Millersville Univ. | Millersville | | X | | | |
| Neumann College | Aston | X | | | | |
| Pennsylvania State Univ. | Univ. Park | X | X | X | | |
| Temple Univ. | Philadelphia | X | X | X | | |
| Thiel College | Greenville | X | X | | | |
| Thomas Jefferson Univ. | Philadelphia | X | X | X | | |
| Univ. of Pennsylvania | Philadelphia | X | X | X | X | X |
| Univ. of Pittsburgh | Pittsburgh | X | X | X | X | |
| Univ. of Scranton | Scranton | X | X | | | |
| Villanova Univ. | Villanova | X | X | X | | |
| Waynesburg College | Waynesburg | X | X | | | |
| West Chester Univ. | West Chester | X | X | | | |
| Widener Univ. | Chester | X | X | X | X | |
| Wilkes College | Wilkes-Barre | X | X | X | | |
| York College of Pennsylvania | York | X | X | | | |

### PUERTO RICO

| Institution and State | City | GN | RN | MS | DC | PD* |
|---|---|---|---|---|---|---|
| Humacao Univ. College | Humacao | X | | | | |
| Univ. of Puerto Rico-Arecibo | Arecibo | X | | | | |
| Univ. of Puerto Rico-Mayaguez | Mayaguez | X | | | | |

(continued)

| Institution and State | City | GN | RN | MS | DC | PD* |
|---|---|---|---|---|---|---|
| **RHODE ISLAND** | | | | | | |
| Rhode Island College | Providence | X | X | | | |
| Salve Regina College | Newport | X | X | | | |
| Univ. of Rhode Island | Kingston | X | X | X | X | |
| **SOUTH CAROLINA** | | | | | | |
| Bob Jones Univ. | Greenville | X | X | | | |
| Clemson Univ. | Clemson | X | X | X | | |
| Lander College | Greenwood | X | | | | |
| Medical Univ. of South Carolina | Charleston | X | X | X | | |
| South Carolina State College | Orangeburg | X | X | | | |
| Univ. of South Carolina | Columbia | X | X | X | X | |
| Univ. of South Carolina at Aiken | Aiken | | X | | | |
| Univ. of South Carolina-Spartanburg | Spartanburg | X | X | | | |
| **SOUTH DAKOTA** | | | | | | |
| Augustana College | Sioux Falls | X | X | | | |
| Mount Marty College | Yankton | X | X | | | |
| South Dakota State Univ. | Brookings | X | X | X | | |
| **TENNESSEE** | | | | | | |
| Austin Peay State Univ. | Clarksville | X | X | | | |
| Belmont College | Nashville | X | | | | |
| Carson-Newman | | | | | | |

(continued)

*Key to Programs Offered: GN = Generic Baccalaureate; RN = RN Baccalaureate; MS = Master's; DC = Doctoral; PD = Postdoctoral

| Institution and State | City | GN | RN | MS | DC | PD* |
|---|---|---|---|---|---|---|
| College | Jefferson City | X | X | | | |
| East Tennessee State Univ. | Johnson City | X | X | | | |
| Lincoln Memorial Univ. | Harrogate | | X | | | |
| Memphis State Univ. | Memphis | X | X | | | |
| Middle Tennessee State Univ. | Murfreesboro | X | | | | |
| Southern Coll. of 7th Day Adventists | Collegedale | | X | | | |
| Tennessee State Univ. | Nashville | X | | | | |
| Tennessee Technological Univ. | Cookeville | X | | | | |
| Union Univ. | Jackson | | X | | | |
| Univ. of Tennessee at Martin | Martin | X | | | | |
| Univ. of Tennessee-Chattanooga | Chattanooga | X | X | | | |
| Univ. of Tennessee-Knoxville | Knoxville | X | | | X | X |
| Univ. of Tennessee-Memphis | Memphis | X | X | X | X | |
| Vanderbilt Univ. | Nashville | | | | X | |

## TEXAS

| Institution and State | City | GN | RN | MS | DC | PD* |
|---|---|---|---|---|---|---|
| Abilene Intercollegiate School | Abilene | X | X | | | |
| Baylor Univ. | Dallas | X | X | | | |
| Corpus Christi State Univ. | Corpus Christi | | X | X | | |
| Dallas Baptist College | Dallas | X | X | | | |
| Houston Baptist Univ. | Houston | X | | | | |

(continued)

| Institution and State | City | GN | RN | MS | DC | PD* |
|---|---|---|---|---|---|---|
| Incarnate Word College | San Antonio | X | X | X | | |
| Midwestern State Univ. | Wichita Falls | X | X | | | |
| Prairie View A & M Univ. | Houston | X | X | | | |
| Southwestern Adventist College | Keene | | X | | | |
| Stephen F. Austin State Univ. | Nacogdoches | X | X | | | |
| Texas Christian Univ. | Fort Worth | X | X | | | |
| Texas Tech Univ. Health Sci. Ctr. | Lubbock | X | X | X | | |
| Texas Woman's Univ. | Denton | X | X | X | X | |
| **Univ. of Texas Health Science Center-Houston** | Houston | X | | X | | |
| Univ. of Texas Health Science Center-San Antonio | San Antonio | X | X | X | | |
| Univ. of Mary Hardin-Baylor | Belton | X | X | | | |
| Univ. of Texas-Arlington | Arlington | X | X | X | | |
| Univ. of Texas-Austin | Austin | X | X | X | X | |
| Univ. of Texas-El Paso | El Paso | X | X | X | | |
| Univ. of Texas-Galveston | Galveston | X | X | X | | |
| Univ. of Texas-Tyler | Tyler | X | X | X | | |
| West Texas State Univ. | Canyon | X | X | X | | |

(*continued*)

*Key to Programs Offered: GN = Generic Baccalaureate; RN = RN Baccalaureate; MS = Master's; DC = Doctoral; PD = Postdoctoral

| Institution and State | City | GN | RN | MS | DC | PD* |
|---|---|---|---|---|---|---|
| **UTAH** | | | | | | |
| Brigham Young Univ. | Provo | X | X | X | | |
| Univ. of Utah | Salt Lake City | X | X | X | X | X |
| Weber State College | Ogden | | X | | | |
| Westminster College | Salt Lake City | X | X | | | |
| **VERMONT** | | | | | | |
| Univ. of Vermont | Burlington | X | X | X | | |
| Vermont College of Norwich Univ. | Montpelier | | X | | | |
| **VIRGIN ISLANDS** | | | | | | |
| Univ. of the Virgin Islands | St. Thomas | X | X | | | |
| **VIRGINIA** | | | | | | |
| Christopher Newport College | Newport News | | X | | | |
| Eastern Mennonite College | Harrisonburg | X | X | | | |
| George Mason Univ. | Fairfax | X | X | X | X | |
| Hampton Univ. | Hampton | X | X | X | | |
| James Madison Univ. | Harrisonburg | X | X | | | |
| Liberty Univ. | Lynchburg | X | X | | | |
| Lynchburg College | Lynchburg | X | X | | | |
| Marymount Univ. | Arlington | | X | X | | |
| Norfolk State Univ. | Norfolk | | X | | | |
| Old Dominion Univ. | Norfolk | X | X | X | | |
| Radford Univ. | Radford | X | X | X | | |
| Shenandoah College & Conservatory | Winchester | | X | | | |
| Univ. of Virginia | Charlottesville | X | X | X | X | |
| Virginia Commonwealth Univ. | Richmond | X | X | X | X | |
| Virginia State Univ. | Petersburg | X | | | | |

(continued)

| Institution and State | City | GN | RN | MS | DC | PD* |
|---|---|---|---|---|---|---|
| **WASHINGTON** | | | | | | |
| Gonzaga Univ. | Spokane | | X | | | |
| Intercollegiate Center for Nursing Research | Spokane | X | X | X | | |
| Pacific Lutheran Univ. | Tacoma | X | X | | | |
| Saint Martin's College | Lacey | | X | | | |
| Seattle Pacific Univ. | Seattle | X | X | X | | |
| Seattle Univ. | Seattle | X | X | | | |
| Univ. of Washington | Seattle | X | X | X | X | X |
| **WEST VIRGINIA** | | | | | | |
| Alderson-Broaddus College | Phillipi | X | X | | | |
| Davis & Elkins College | Elkins | | X | | | |
| Marshall Univ. | Huntington | X | X | | | |
| Shepherd College | Shepherdstown | X | X | | | |
| Univ. of Charleston | Charleston | X | X | | | |
| West Liberty State College | West Liberty | X | X | | | |
| West Virginia Univ. | Morgantown | X | X | X | | |
| West Virginia Wesleyan College | Buckhannon | X | X | | | |
| Wheeling College | Wheeling | X | X | | | |
| **WISCONSIN** | | | | | | |
| Alverno College | Milwaukee | X | X | | | |
| Carroll College | Milwaukee | X | X | | | |
| Concordia Univ. Wisconsin | Mequon | X | X | | | |
| Edgewood College | Madison | X | X | | | |
| Marian College of Fond du Lac | Fond du Lac | X | X | | | |

(continued)

*Key to Programs Offered: **GN** = Generic Baccalaureate; **RN** = RN Baccalaureate; **MS** = Master's; **DC** = Doctoral; **PD** = Postdoctoral

| Institution and State | City | GN | RN | MS | DC | PD* |
|---|---|---|---|---|---|---|
| Marquette Univ. | Milwaukee | X | X | X | | |
| Mount Senario College | Ladysmith | | X | | | |
| Silver Lake College | Manitowoc | | X | | | |
| Univ. of Wisconsin-Eau Claire | Eau Claire | X | X | X | | |
| Univ. of Wisconsin-Green Bay | Green Bay | | X | | | |
| Univ. of Wisconsin-Madison | Madison | X | | X | X | |
| Univ. of Wisconsin-Milwaukee | Milwaukee | X | X | X | X | |
| Univ. of Wisconsin-Oshkosh | Oshkosh | X | X | X | | |
| Viterbo College | LaCrosse | X | X | | | |

## WYOMING

| | | | | | | |
|---|---|---|---|---|---|---|
| Univ. of Wyoming | Laramie | X | X | X | | |

# INFORMATION WAS NOT AVAILABLE ON THE FOLLOWING INSTITUTIONS (1/10/90)

| Institution and State | City |
|---|---|

## ALABAMA

| | |
|---|---|
| Birmingham South-ern College | Birmingham |
| Mobile College | Mobile |

## CALIFORNIA

| | |
|---|---|
| Biola Univ. | La Mirada |
| Cal. State Univ.-Dominguez Hills | Carson |
| California State Univ.-Hayward | Hayward |

*(continued)*

## Institution and State        City

Pacific Union
College                 Los Angeles
Point Loma College      San Diego

## COLORADO

Regis College           Denver
Univ. of Southern
Colorado                Pueblo

## CONNECTICUT

Central Connecticut
State Univ.             New Britain

## DISTRICT OF COLUMBIA

Univ. of the District
of Columbia             Washington

## FLORIDA

Florida A & M
Univ.                   Tallahassee

## GEORGIA

Columbus College        Columbus
Morris Brown
College                 Atlanta
West Georgia
College                 Carrollton

## ILLINOIS

Southern Illinois
Univ.                   Edwardsville

## INDIANA

Marian College          Indianapolis

## IOWA

Iowa Wesleyan
College                 Mount Pleasant
Marycrest College       Davenport

(continued)

## Institution and State — City

### KENTUCKY

| | |
|---|---|
| Bellarmine College | Louisville |
| Eastern Kentucky Univ. | Richmond |
| Murray State Univ. | Murray |

### LOUISIANA

| | |
|---|---|
| Dillard Univ. | New Orleans |
| Grambling State Univ. | Grambling |
| Nicholls State Univ. | Thibodaux |
| Northwestern State Univ. | Shreveport |
| William Carey College | New Orleans |

### MAINE

| | |
|---|---|
| Westbrook College | Portland |

### MARYLAND

| | |
|---|---|
| Bowie State College | Bowie |

### MASSACHUSETTS

| | |
|---|---|
| Simmons College | Boston |
| Stonehill College | North Easton |
| Worcester State College | Worcester |

### MICHIGAN

| | |
|---|---|
| Andrews Univ. | Berrien Springs |
| Univ. of Detroit | Detroit |

### MINNESOTA

| | |
|---|---|
| Mankato State Univ. | Mankato |

### MISSOURI

| | |
|---|---|
| Hannibal-LaGrange College | Hannibal |

(continued)

| Institution and State | City |
|---|---|
| Missouri Baptist College | St. Louis |

## NEW HAMPSHIRE

| | |
|---|---|
| Colby-Sawyer College | New London |
| Rivier College | Nashua |

## NEW JERSEY

| | |
|---|---|
| Bloomfield College | Bloomfield |
| Univ. of Medicine & Dentistry of NJ | Newark |

## NEW YORK

| | |
|---|---|
| College of Staten Island | Staten Island |
| Mercy College | Dobbs Ferry |
| St. Joseph's College | Brooklyn |
| Wagner College | Staten Island |

## NORTH CAROLINA

| | |
|---|---|
| Atlantic Christian College | Wilson |
| Methodist College | Fayetteville |
| Wingate College | Wingate |

## NORTH DAKOTA

| | |
|---|---|
| Dickinson State College | Dickinson |
| Univ. of Mary | Bismarck |

## OHIO

| | |
|---|---|
| Franciscan Univ. of Steubenville | Steubenville |
| Kent State Univ. | Kent |
| Malone College | Canton |
| Miami Univ. | Hamilton |
| Otterbein College | Westerville |

*(continued)*

| Institution and State | City |
|---|---|

**OKLAHOMA**

| | |
|---|---|
| Oklahoma Baptist Univ. | Shawnee |

**OREGON**

| | |
|---|---|
| Southern Oregon State College | Ashland |

**PENNSYLVANIA**

| | |
|---|---|
| Clarion State College | Oil City |
| College Misericordia | Dallas |
| Saint Francis College | Loretto |
| Slippery Rock Univ. | Slippery Rock |

**PUERTO RICO**

| | |
|---|---|
| Antillian College | Mayaquez |
| Caribbean Univ. College | Bayamon |
| Catholic Univ. of Puerto Rico | Ponce |
| InterAmerican Univ. of Puerto Rico | Hato Rey |
| Univ. of Puerto Rico | San Juan |

**TEXAS**

| | |
|---|---|
| Angelo State Univ. | San Angelo |
| Lamar Univ. | Beaumont |
| Pan American Univ. | Edinburg |

**VERMONT**

| | |
|---|---|
| Castleton State College | Castleton |

**VIRGINIA**

| | |
|---|---|
| Averett College | Danville |
| City Univ. | Bellevue |

(continued)

## Institution and State        City

**WASHINGTON**

City University        Bellevue

**WEST VIRGINIA**

Salem College        Salem

**WISCONSIN**

Cardinal Stritch
College        Milwaukee

# Index